W9-CBM-830

Tarascon Pediatric Emergency Pocketbook

4ᵗʰ Edition. From the publishers of the *Tarascon Pocket Pharmacopoeia*.

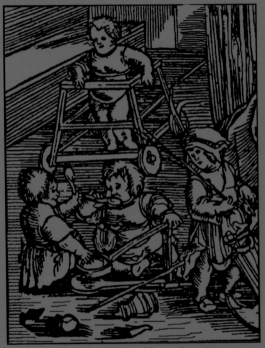

Steven G Rothrock, MD

Tarascon Pediatric Emergency Pocketbook, 4th Edition

SEE PAGE 192 FOR ORDERING INFORMATION

ABBREVIATIONS		g	grams	m²	square meter	PPV	+pressure
bid	twice per day	h	hour	mEq	milliequiv		ventilation
BP	blood pressure	Hb	hemoglobin	min	minute	PR	by rectum
cm	centimeters	HR	heart rate	ml	milliliters	prn	as needed
CNS	central nervous sys	ICP	intracranial	mo	month	qd	every day
CSF	cerebrospinal fluid		pressure	NS	normal	qid	4 times/day
d	day	IM	intramuscular		saline	SC	subcutaneous
D₅W	5% dextrose in H₂0	IO	intraosseous	O₂	oxygen	SL	sublingual
ET	endotracheal	IV	intravenous	OD	overdose	tid	3 times/day
F	French	J	joules	PO	by mouth	µg	micrograms
fx	fracture	kg	kilograms	PMN	neutrophil	y	years old

Tarascon Publishing, PO Box 1159, Loma Linda, California 92354

Important Caution - Please Read This!

The information in *Pediatric Emergency Pocketbook* is compiled from sources believed to be reliable, and exhaustive efforts have been put forth to make the book as accurate as possible. *However the accuracy and completeness of this work cannot be guaranteed.* Despite our best efforts this book may contain typographical errors and omissions. The *Pediatric Emergency Pocketbook* is intended as a quick and convenient reminder of information you have already learned elsewhere. The contents are to be used as a guide only, and health care professionals should use sound clinical judgment and individualize therapy to each specific patient care situation. This book is not meant to be a replacement for training, experience, continuing medical education, or studying the latest drug prescribing literature. This book is sold without warranties of any kind, express or implied. The publisher & editors disclaim any liability, loss, or damage caused by the contents. *If you do not wish to be bound by the foregoing cautions & conditions, you may return your undamaged book for a full refund.*

The Tarascon Pediatric Emergency Pocketbook, 4ᵗʰ Ed

ISBN 1-882742-28-1. Copyright © 1995,1997,1999, 2003 Mako Publishing, Inc, Winter Park, Florida. Printed in the USA. All rights reserved. Published & marketed under exclusive license to Tarascon Publishing (Tarascon Inc, Loma Linda, CA). No portion of this publication may be reproduced or stored in a retrieval system in any form or by any means (including electronic, mechanical, photocopying, etc.) without prior written permission from us. We welcome suggestions for improving this book. The cover is a detail from the woodcut *"Of a fruitful and well-spoken housewife"*, Francesco Petrarcas, Germany, 1620.

EDITORS: Steven G. Rothrock MD, FACEP, FAAP; Associate Professor, Emergency Medicine, Orlando, FL **Steven M. Green MD**, FACEP; Professor Emergency Medicine, EM. Residency Director,Loma Linda University School of Medicine, Loma Linda, CA
EDITORIAL BOARD: Mark C Clark MD FAAP, FACEP; Associate Professor University of Florida, College of Medicine. **Daniel C Farrell MD** Fellow Pediatric Orthopedics, Denver Children's Hospital, CO **Daniel Isaacman MD**, FAAP; Assoc Professor Emergency Medicine Eastern Virginia Med. School, Director, Peds EM, Children's Hosp. of the King's Daughter. **Chris King MD**, FACEP, Assoc Prof Emerg Med, University of Pittsburgh School of Medicine, PA **Angela McQueen PharmD** Clin Pharmacy Consultant, Partners Comm. Healthcare, Inc, Needham, MA, **Larry Mellick MD**, FAAP, FACEP; Professor Emerg Medicine, Chairman, Emergency Medicine, Medical College Georgia, Augusta, GA

Abuse (Non-Accidental Trauma)

Appearance of Cutaneous Bruises Over Time[1]	0 - 2 days	swollen, tender, red, blue, purple
	3 - 6 days	blue, green
	6 - 10 days	green, brown
	10 - 14 days	tan, yellow
	14 - 30 days	faded to clear

[1]Dating bruises based on color can be inaccurate and ages are only a rough estimate.
Note: any bite marks with distance between incisors > 3 cm was made by an adult.

Bony Injuries Associated with Child Abuse

Fractures Associated With a High or Moderate Risk of Abuse	• Fractures in different stages of healing or delayed presentation
	• Fractures inconsistent with history or development of child
	• Metaphyseal-epiphyseal fractures (e.g. corner, bucket handle, and metaphyseal lucency)
	• Posterior rib fractures, Scapular fractures, Sternal fractures
	• Avulsion fractures of the clavicle or acromion process
	• Skull – if multiple, depressed, or across suture line
	• Pelvic or spinal fractures without significant force
	• Spinous process, vertebral body fractures (70% anterosuperior or superior end plate ± compression) and subluxations
	• Femur fractures ≤ 1-2 years old
	• Non-supracondylar humerus fracture
Fractures Associated With a Low Risk of Abuse	• Clavicle fractures (except avulsion fractures)
	• Distal tibia spiral fractures (Toddler's fracture) unless non-ambulatory infant
	• Supracondylar fractures, fractures of the hand or feet (except digital fractures in non-ambulatory infants)
	• Torus fractures of long bones

Pediatr Emerg Med Reports 1998; 3: 1; & 2001 6: 57.

Appearance of Fractures Over Time	4-10 days	Resolution of soft tissue swelling
	10-14 days	New periosteal bone
	14-21 days	Fracture line definition lost & Soft callus present
	21-42 days	Hard callus present
	3-24 months	Remodeling of fracture

Beaty/Kasser (eds) *Fractures in Children* Lippincott, 2001

See page 165 for Differentiation of Head Injury due to Accidental from Head Injury due to Non-accidental Trauma.

Non-Bony Injuries Associated with Abuse

CNS	• Interhemispheric falx bleed (highly specific), subdural hematoma (common – less specific), basal ganglia edema, large extra-axial fluid (old trauma)
Ophthalmologic	• Retinal hemorrhage with macular folds, vitreous bleed
ENT & Oral	• Buccal, palatal, gingival contusions, frenulum tear • Petechiae along inner/outer ear helix ("tin ear syndrome": ear injury with ipsilateral brain injury & retinal hemorrhage)
Abdomen/GI	• Duodenal/jejunal perf., left lobe liver/pancreatic injury
Skin	• Burns: stocking/glove, genital, axillary, posterior thorax • Bruises: on face, back, abdomen, buttocks, nonexposed body areas (axillae, neck, genitalia). Injuries may be in shape of object inflicting trauma.

Pediatr Radiol 1997; 743; & 2000; 74.

Components of Skeletal Survey[1]	• Skull, Chest, Pelvis, (AP[2] & lateral views) • Lateral spine radiography (lumbar & cervical) • Extremity AP[2] radiography (humeri, forearms, hands [PA, oblique], femurs, tibia/fibula, feet)

[1] Primarily indicated < 2 years old, with more selective use from 2-5 years.
[2] AP – anterior-posterior film   *Pediatrics* 2000; 105: 1345.

Conditions Mimicking Abuse
(Causing Skin[1] or Bony[2] Abnormalities Similar to Abuse)

Bone[2]	• Primary or metastatic tumors, osteomyelitis
Collagen-Vascular[2]	• Ehlers Danlos - *hypermobile joints, skin laxity* • Osteogenesis Imperfecta - *blue sclera, family history, hearing impaired > age 10, yellow-brown/gray teeth enamel fracture, short stature. Radiographs ± osteopenia, thin cortex, bowing or angulation healed fractures, Wormian bones on skull film. 84-95% have abnormal collagen in skin fibroblast studies.*
Hematology[1]	• Leukemia, neuroblastoma, ITP, hemophilia, platelet disorders
Medication[1]	• Prostaglandin E, methotrexate, salicylates, rodenticides
Metabolic[2]	• Copper or calcium deficiency, vitamin C or D deficiency
Skin[1]	• Bullous impetigo, hair tourniquets, cultural dermabrasion (cupping, spooning, coin rubbing), Mongolian spots, epidermolysis bullosa
Vascular[1]	• Henoch Schonlein purpura, erythema multiforme

Age Based Estimates for Vital Signs and Weight (*BP - mean ± 2 standard deviations*)

AGE	Weight(kg)	Heart rate	Resp Rate	Systolic BP	Diastolic BP
premature	1	145/min	~40	42 ± 10	21 ± 8
premature	1-2	135	~40	50 ± 10	28 ± 8
newborn	2-3	125	~40	60 ± 10	37 ± 8
1 month	4	120	24-35	80 ± 16	46 ± 16
6 month	7	130	24-35	89 ± 29	60 ± 10
1 year	10	120	20-30	96 ± 30	66 ± 25
2-3 years	12-14	115	20-30	99 ± 25	64 ± 25
4-5 years	16-18	100	20-30	99 ± 20	65 ± 20
6-8 years	20-26	100	12-25	100 ± 15	60 ± 10
10-12 yr	32-42	75	12-25	110 ± 17	60 ± 10
>14 yr	>50	70	12-18	118 ± 20	60 ± 10

Resuscitation Equipment / 1st Dose of Drugs Based on Length, Weight, or Age

Length (cm)	58-70	70-85	85-95	95-107	107-124	124-138	138-156
Weight (kg)	5-7	8-11	12-14	15-17	18-24	25-32	33-40
Age (years)	0.5	1	2	3	5	8-10	>12
Bag mask	infant	child	child	child	child	child/adult	adult
Oral airway	infant	small child	child	child	child	small adult	adult
Laryngeal mask	1	2	2	2	2.5	2.5-3	3
Oxygen mask	newborn	peds	peds	peds	adult	adult	adult
ET Tube	3.0/3.5	3.5/4.0	4.0/4.5	4.5	5.0	5.5	6.0
Laryngoscope	1 Miller	1 Miller	2 Miller	2[a]	2[a]	2-3[a]	3[a]
Suction catheter	8F	8-10F	10F	10F	10F	10F	12F
Stylet	6F	6F	6F	6F	14F	14F	14F
Nasogastric tube	5-8F	8-10F	10F	10-12F	12-14F	14-18F	18F
Urine Catheter	5-8F	8-10F	10F	10-12F	10-12F	12-14F	16F
Chest Tube	10-12F	16-20F	20-24F	20-24F	24-32F	28-32F	32-40F
amiodarone	25-35	40-55	60-70	75-85	90-120	125-150	150
ampicillin	250-350	400-550	600-700	750-850	900-1200	1250-1600	1650-2000
atropine	0.1-0.14	0.16-0.22	0.24-0.28	0.3-0.34	0.36-0.48	0.5-0.64	0.66-0.80
bicarb (mEq)	5-7	8-11	12-14	15-17	18-24	25-32	33-40
ceftriaxone	250-350	400-550	600-700	750-850	900-1200	1250-1600	1650-2000
cefotaxime	250-350	400-550	600-700	750-850	900-1200	1250-1600	1650-2000
defibrillation (J)	10-14	16-22	24-28	30-34	36-48	50-64	66-80
dextrose (g)	5-7	8-11	12-14	15-17	18-24	25-32	33-40
diazepam	0.5-2.1	0.8-3.3	1.2-4.2	1.5-5.1	1.8-7	2.5-9	3.3-10
epinephrine	0.05-.07	0.08-0.11	0.12-0.14	0.15-0.17	0.18-0.24	0.25-0.32	0.33-0.40
lidocaine	5-7	8-11	12-14	15-17	18-24	25-32	33-40
mannitol (g)	5-7	8-11	12-14	15-17	18-24	25-32	33-40
midazolam	0.5-.7	0.8-1.1	1.2-1.4	1.5-1.7	1.8-2.4	2.5-3.2	3.3-4
normal saline[b]	100-140	160-220	240-280	300-340	360-480	500-640	660-800
succinylcholine	10-14	16-22	24-28	30-34	36-48	50-64	66-80

All drugs are in mg unless otherwise specified. [a]Miller or Macintosh. [b]Bolus (ml) for hypovolemia.

CPR Maneuvers and Techniques In Newborns, Infants, & Children

Maneuver	Newly born/Neonate	Infant(<1 year)	Child (1-8 years)
Open Airway	Head tilt-chin lift (jaw lift if trauma) – all ages		
Breathing	May require 30-40	Two breaths at	Two breaths at
Initial	cm H_2O pressure	1-1.5 sec/breath	1-1.5 sec/breath
Subsequent	30-60 breaths/min	20 breaths/min	20 breaths/min
Circulation*			
Check pulse	Umbilical/brachial	Brachial or femoral	Carotid
Compress at	Lower ½ sternum	Lower ½ sternum	Lower ½ sternum
Compress with	Two thumbs encircle chest with hands	Two thumbs encircle chest with hands	Heel of one hand
Depth	One third to one half depth of chest for all listed ages		
*Rate***	120/min @ 3:1	at least 100/min 5:1	100/min @ 5:1
Ratio	3:1 (interpose breaths)	5:1 (interpose breaths)	5:1 (interpose breaths)
Airway Obstruction	Back blows Chest thrusts	Back blows Chest thrusts	Abd or chest thrust or back blow,

*Also check for normal breathing, movement, or coughing. Lay people do not check pulse
** Total number of events - compressions plus breaths

Newly Born Resuscitation

Birth

• Clear of meconium? • Breathing or crying? • Color pink, or term delivery?	**Yes to all** →	Routine care • Provide warmth & dry • Clear airway

No

• Provide warmth, position/clear airway (if meconium see page 7)
• Dry, stimulate, reposition and provide O_2 prn

• Evaluate respirations, heart rate (HR) and color	**Breathing, pink & HR > 100**	Supportive care

Apnea or HR < 100

• Positive pressure ventilation	**Ventilating, pink & HR > 100**	Ongoing care

HR < 60 ↓   ↑ HR > 60

• Positive pressure ventilation[1]
• Chest compressions

[1] consider endotracheal intubation if + pressure ventilation ineffective here

• Epinephrine IV/IO/ET/Umbilical vein[1] 0.01- 0.03 mg/kg (0.1-0.3 ml/kg of 1:10,000) q 3-5 min

Size of Endotracheal Tube/Laryngoscope Blade for Newly Born

Gestational age	Birth weight (g)	Size of ET Tube[1,2]	Blade size[3]
<28 weeks	<1,000	2.5	Number 0 straight
28-34 weeks	1,000-2,000	2.5-3.0	Number 0 straight
34-38 weeks	2,000-3,000	3.0-3.5	Number 0 straight
>38 weeks	Term (>3,000)	3.5-4.0	Number 1 straight

[1]Internal diameter in millimeters, [2]Depth at gum line = 6 + newly born weight in kg
[3] Wide/fat straight blades (e.g. Wis-Hipple, Flagg) may be superior to thin (Miller) blades for manipulating normally large neonatal/infant tongues

Normal Blood Pressure for Different Birth Weights

Weight	<1 kg	1-2 kg	2-3 kg	>3 kg
Systolic BP	40-60	50-60	50-70	50-80
Diastolic BP	15-35	20-40	25-45	30-50

Meconium Management

Intrapartum - As soon as head delivered (before body delivered), suction, mouth, pharynx and nose with large bore suction catheter (12-14 F) or bulb syringe.
Following delivery – Perform immediate direct laryngoscopy with suctioning ONLY if (1) ↓ respirations (2) ↓ muscle tone or (3) HR < 100 beats/minute. Repeat until little meconium is recovered or HR < 60-80 (indicating need for resuscitation). Perform tracheal suctioning before initiating positive pressure ventilation (PPV). If patient becomes severely distressed, positive pressure ventilation may be required even if all of meconium is not suctioned out.

Apgar Scoring

Sign	0	1	2
Heart rate	absent	<100	>100
Respiratory effort	absent	slow / irregular	good, cry
Muscle tone	flaccid	some extremity flexion	active motion
Reflex irritability	no response	grimace	vigorous cry
Color	pale	cyanotic	completely pink

Abnormal Glucose for Neonates

Administer glucose to all neonates with bedside glucose <50 mg/dl, as this test may be inaccurate below this level.

Age	Hypoglycemia
premature	<25
full term <72h	<35
full term >72h	<45

Normal Arterial Blood/Hct Values in Full Term Newly Born

Age	PaO2	PaCO2	pH	Base excess	Hct (vol %)
1 hour	63 mmHg	36 mmHg	7.33	- 6.0 mEq/L	53
24 hours	73 mmHg	33 mmHg	7.37	- 5.0 mEq/L	55

DRUG THERAPY: IO route can be used for therapy if IV, umbilical vein unavailable.

Epinephrine – Indicated If HR < 60 after 30 seconds of ventilation and CPR. Dose at 0.01-0.03 mg/kg IV/IO/ET/Umbilical vein (0.1-0.3 ml/kg of 1:10,000). Repeat q 3-5 minuntes prn.

Dopamine – Use if unresponsive hypotension. See page 191 for infusion.

Glucose: Hypoglycemia is most common in premature or small for gestational age infants following a prolonged and difficult labor, mothers on ritodrine or terbutaline, and infants of diabetics. Hypoxia, hypothermia, hyperthermia and sepsis deplete glucose stores. Treat with 1-2 ml/kg of $D_{10}W$ IV push, then infuse 6-8 mg/kg/min.

Naloxone: 0.1 mg/kg IV/ET/Umbilical vein/IM/SC if severe respiratory depression & maternal narcotic administration in prior 4 hours. Caution: naloxone may precipitate seizures if mother used narcotics chronically.

Sodium bicarbonate: 1-2 mEq/L IV/Umbilical vein of 0.5 mEq/L solution over ≥ 2 minutes. IV push may cause venous irritation/CNS bleeding. Not routinely used.

Volume: NS, LR or O neg blood as needed at 10 ml/kg IV/Umbilical over 5-10 min.

Umbilical Artery/Vein Catheterization

Umbilical vein is single thin walled vessel that is the preferred access site during newly born resuscitation. Prep abdomen/cord sterilely, loosely tie umbilical tape to cord base for anchoring/hemostasis. Cut cord with scalpel 2 cm from abdomen wall. **Umbilical vein:** remove visible clot, flush catheter with heparin. Use 3.5-4 French (Fr) catheter if < 2 kg and 5-8 Fr for > 2 kg neonates. Advance umbilical catheter (5-8 Fr) through vein until blood return or 4-5 cm. Lateral clavicle to umbilicus length X 0.6 places catheter tip above diaphragm. Tighten umbilical tape to secure, and withdraw after resuscitation.

Umbilical artery: after dilating with iris forcep, insert tip of catheter to lumen. (1) ideally use nomogram with total body length to estimate depth **OR** (2) for thoracic umbilical artery catheter – estimate shoulder to umbilicus (S-U) distance. If (S-U) < 13 cm, insert S-U distance + 1 cm. If S-U > 13 cm, insert to depth of S-U distance + 2 cm. **OR** (3) Estimated depth of low UA catheter: [Birth weight (kg) + 7] cm.

Intraosseous (IO)

Place IO in proximal tibia (1-2 cm distal + medial to tuberosity), distal tibia (medial malleolus - tibial shaft junction), or distal femur (as condyle tapers into shaft). After local anesthetic, & site sterilized, puncture skin, direct needle away from growth plate. Push and rotate gently until "pop" and advance 0.5-1 cm. Confirm by (1) aspiration of marrow, OR (2) easy infusion of 3 ml NS with aspiration of injected fluid that returns with pink tinge. Aspirate for labs (Hb, T & C, electrolytes, BUN, creatinine, NOT white cell count, NOT platelets) & infuse medications/fluid/blood with large syringe. Any advanced life support drug or blood can be given IO. Watch for leak. Remove as soon as alternate access site is obtained.

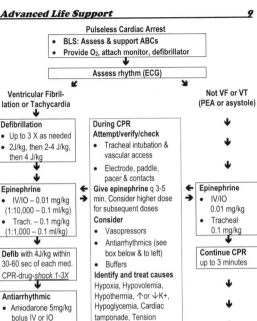

Pulseless Cardiac Arrest

- BLS: Assess & support ABCs
- Provide O₂, attach monitor, defibrillator

Assess rhythm (ECG)

Ventricular Fibrillation or Tachycardia | **Not VF or VT (PEA or asystole)**

Defibrillation
- Up to 3 X as needed
- 2J/kg, then 2-4 J/kg, then 4 J/kg

During CPR
Attempt/verify/check
- Tracheal intubation & vascular access
- Electrode, paddle, pacer & contacts

Give epinephrine q 3-5 min. Consider higher dose for subsequent doses

Consider
- Vasopressors
- Antiarrhythmics (see box below & to left)
- Buffers

Identify and treat causes
Hypoxia, Hypovolemia, Hypothermia, ↑or ↓K+, Hypoglycemia, Cardiac tamponade, Tension Pneumothorax, Toxins, Thromboembolism

Epinephrine
- IV/IO – 0.01 mg/kg (1:10,000 – 0.1 ml/kg)
- Trach. – 0.1 mg/kg (1:1,000 – 0.1 ml/kg)

Epinephrine
- IV/IO 0.01 mg/kg
- Tracheal 0.1 mg/kg

Defib with 4J/kg within 30-60 sec of each med. CPR-*drug-shock 1-3X*

Continue CPR up to 3 minutes

Antiarrhythmic
- Amiodarone 5mg/kg bolus IV or IO
- Lidocaine 1 mg/kg bolus IV/IO/ET
- Mg 25-50 mg/kg IV or IO if torsades or ↓ Mg (magnesium)

Reassess rhythm

Attempt defibrillation with 4 J/kg within 30-60 seconds of each medication (CPR – Drug – *Shock 1 to 3 times*)

Vascular Access

See page 8 for techniques of umbilical vein/artery, and intraosseous access.

Central Venous Catheter Diameter Based on Age & Site (int. diameter-French [F])	Age (years)	Internal jugular vein	Subclavian vein	Femoral vein
	0 - 0.5	3 F	3 F	3 F
	0.5 - 2	3 F	3 F	3 - 4 F
	3 - 6	4 F	4 F	4 F
	7 - 12	4 - 5 F	4 - 5 F	4 - 5 F

Right Internal Jugular and Right Subclavian (SC) Central Venous Catheter Depth (cm)[1,2]

Initial Catheter Insertion based on Patient Height/Length	Height < 100 cm	Height $100 \geq$ cm
	Initial Catheter Depth = Height (cm)/10 – 1 cm	Initial Catheter Depth = Height (cm)/10 – 2 cm

Initial Catheter Insertion based on Patient Weight (note – chart and formula are based on patient's weight when known and age is only approximated based on patient weight)	Approx. Age	Weight (kg)	Length/Depth(cm)
	0 - 2 mo	3.0 - 4.9	5
	> 2 – 5 mo	5.0 – 6.9	6
	6 – 11 mo	7.0 – 9.9	7
	1 - 2 y	10.0 - 12.9	8
	>2 – 6 y	13.0 - 19.9	9
	>6 – 9 y	20 – 29.9	10
	>9 – 12 y	30 – 39.9	11
	> 12 – 14 y	40-50	12

[1] If < 100cm, skin for SC vein punctured 1 cm lateral to midclavicle, 2 cm lateral if > 100 cm
[2] Anesth Analg 2001; 93: 883. Formulas will place 97-98% of catheters above right atrium

Femoral Vein Catheter Mean Length/Insertion Depth

Age	Weight (kg)	Height (cm)	Length (cm)	Age	Weight (kg)	Height (cm)	Length (cm)
1 mo	4.2	55	15.7	2 y	12.8	88	24.2
3 mo	5.8	61	17.3	4 y	16.5	103	28.1
6 mo	7.8	68	19.1	6 y	20.5	116	31.4
9 mo	9.2	72	20.1	8 y	26	127	34.2
1 y	10.2	76	21.1	10 y	31	137	36.8
1.5 y	11.5	83	22.9	12 y	39	149	39.9

Airway Management

<table>
<tr><td></td><td>Age</td><td>Weight (kg)</td><td>ET Tube[1]</td><td>Laryngoscope[2]</td></tr>
<tr><td rowspan="15">Endotracheal Tube and Blade Size</td><td>premature</td><td>1.5</td><td>2.5 - 3.0</td><td>straight 0</td></tr>
<tr><td>term</td><td>3.0</td><td>3.0 - 3.5</td><td>straight 0-1</td></tr>
<tr><td>3 months</td><td>5.5</td><td>3.5 - 4.0</td><td>straight 1</td></tr>
<tr><td>6 months</td><td>7</td><td>3.5-4.0</td><td>straight 1</td></tr>
<tr><td>1 year</td><td>10</td><td>4.0-4.5</td><td>straight 1</td></tr>
<tr><td>2 years</td><td>12</td><td>4.0-4.5</td><td>straight 1</td></tr>
<tr><td>3 years</td><td>14</td><td>5.0</td><td>Miller/Macintosh 2</td></tr>
<tr><td>4 years</td><td>16</td><td>5.5</td><td>Miller/Macintosh 2</td></tr>
<tr><td>5 years</td><td>18</td><td>5.5</td><td>Miller/Macintosh 2</td></tr>
<tr><td>6-7 years</td><td>20-22</td><td>6.0</td><td>Miller/Macintosh 2</td></tr>
<tr><td>8-10 years</td><td>25-30</td><td>6.0 - 6.5</td><td>Miller/Macintosh 2</td></tr>
<tr><td>10-12 years</td><td>30-35</td><td>6.5</td><td>Miller/Macintosh 2</td></tr>
<tr><td>12-14 years</td><td>35-40</td><td>7.0</td><td>Miller/Macintosh 3</td></tr>
</table>

[1] Internal diameter in millimeters, [2] Wide/fat straight blades (Wis-Hipple, Flagg) may be superior to thin (Miller) blades for manipulating normally large tongues in infants < 2 yo.

Formula for estimating ET tube size based on age

- Tube internal diameter estimate (mm) = [16 + age in years] ÷ 4. Note in table above that this formula may slightly overestimate tube size if < 2 years old.
- Use uncuffed ET tubes under age 8.
- If cuffed subtract 0.5 mm from size estimate.
- See page 5 & above for age, length/weight based estimate for ET tube & meds.

Anatomic Indicators of Difficult Pediatric Airway

- *Oropharyngeal exam* - inability to visualize tonsillar pillars, soft palate, or uvula
- *Atlanto-occipital joint* - extension less than 35 degrees
- *Thyromental distance* - distance > 2 adult fingerwidths (3 cm) from mandibular ramus to the thyroid cartilage in an adolescent or child **Or** more than 1 adult fingerwidth (1.5 cm) in infant. Measure with neck in neutral position.
- *Temporomandibular joint* - limited hinge movement of temporomandibular joint (e.g. juvenile rheumatoid arthritis, scoliosis, inflammatory trismus from deep space infection, or mandibular fracture)
- *Congenital airway anomalies* - cleft palate, maxillary or mandibular anomalies, micrognathia, macroglossia, glossoptosis.
- *Maxillary abnormality* - protruding maxillary incisors or maxillofacial trauma
- *Upper airway swelling/obstruction* - bleeding, infection, burn, or inhalation injury

Steps for Rapid Sequence Intubation

Equipment
- ready 2 wall suction devices with Yankauer tips, check laryngoscope lights
- appropriate size ET tube and back-up 0.5 to 1 size smaller, consider stylet
- check integrity of inflatable cuff, if present (no cuff if ≤ 8 years of age)

Patient Preparation
- raise bed to comfortable height (e.g., patient's nose at intubator's xiphoid)
- prepare alternate airway plan: transtracheal jet ventilation, cricothyrotomy (>8y)
- estimate patient's weight (e.g., Broselow tape)
- confirm working pulse oximeter and cardiac monitor
- specify personnel for (1) cricoid pressure, (2) neck immobilization if trauma, (3) handling ET tube, (4) watching O_2 sat & cardiac monitors, and (5) medications
- position head appropriately (sniffing position if no trauma)
- draw up all drugs in syringes and ensure secure IV access is available
- preoxygenate with 100% oxygen for at least 3-4 minutes (if time permits)
- perform Sellick maneuver (cricoid pressure)

Medication
- lidocaine 1.5 mg/kg IV if head injured (to attenuate rise in intracranial pressure)
- atropine 0.02 mg/kg IV (min dose 0.1 mg) if < 5 yo (some only use ≤ 1 yo)
- consider use of defasciculating agent IV if > 5 yo (then wait 1.5 to 2 minutes)
- administer sedating and paralyzing agent IV

Drugs for Rapid Sequence Intubation

Agent	Dose IV (mg/kg)	Onset (min)	Key Properties
Defasciculating drug[1]			may occasionally cause paralysis
pancuronium	0.01	3	histamine release, tachycardia
rocuronium	0.06	2-3	
succinylcholine	0.1	3	fasciculations, ↑BP,ICP,GI,eye pressure
vecuronium	0.01	3	minimal tachycardia
Sedating drug			
etomidate	0.3-0.4	1-2	minimal blood pressure effect
fentanyl	2-6 µg/kg	1-2	↑ ICP, chest wall rigidity
ketamine	1-2	< 1	↑ BP, ↑ICP, ↑ GI and eye pressure
midazolam	0.1-0.2	1-3	hypotension
propofol	1.0-2.5	< 1	hypotension
thiopental	2-4	< 1	hypotension, bronchospasm
Paralyzing drug			
succinylcholine[2]	1-2	<1	fasciculations ↑BP,ICP,GI,eye pressures
rocuronium	0.6-1.2	0.5-1.5	rapid onset, short duration (25-60 min)
vecuronium	0.1 - 0.2	1-4	prolonged action

[1]Defasciculation is unnecessary < 5 years (some experts omit in all patients)
[2]Use 2 mg/kg if <10 kg, & 1.5 mg/kg if defasciculating agent used.

Steps to Perform after Intubation	• Check tube placement (breath sounds, CO_2 detector) • Inflate cuff (if present) then release cricoid pressure • Measure and record tube depth (see below) • Reassess patient's clinical status • Obtain CXR to verify correct placement depth • Consider longer-acting sedative and paralytics

Formulas for Estimating Depth of ET tube after Intubation

• Distance in cm from midtrachea to incisors/gum line = 3 x (ET tube ID[1])
• Distance in cm from midtrachea to incisors/gum line = 12 + (age in years)/2
• Distance in cm from midtrachea to incisors/gum line = (height in cm)/10 + 5
• Distance in cm from midtrachea to nares (for nasotracheal) = 12 + (age in y)/2

[1]ID - internal diameter in mm

Laryngeal Mask Airway Sizes

Mask Size	Patient weight	Internal diameter (mm)	cuff volume (ml)
1	< 6.5 kg	5.25	2 - 5
2	6.5 - 20 kg	7	7 - 10
2.5	20 - 30 kg	8.4	14
3	30 - 70 kg	10	15 - 20
4	70 - 90 kg	12	25 - 30
5	> 90 kg	11.5	30 - 40

Rescue Procedure for Transtracheal Jet Ventilation

Place a 14-gauge IV catheter attached to 5ml syringe through cricothyroid membrane. Remove needle, leaving catheter and confirm placement by aspirating air. Attach 3.0 mm ET tube adapter to IV catheter, or attach 3 ml locking syringe (without plunger) to 3 mm ET tube adapter. Attach 10-50 psi 100% O_2 source and deliver O_2 at 20 bursts/minute with inspiratory to expiratory ratio of 1:2 or 1:3.

	Age	Initial PSI	Tidal Volume (ml)
Parameters for transtracheal jet ventilation	< 5 years	5	100
	5-8 years	5-10	240-340
	8-12 years	10-25	340-625
	> 12 years	30-50	700-1000

Guidelines for Mechanical Ventilation

Item	Neonates & Infants	Older Children
Ventilator	pressure-limited if weight <10 kg	volume-limited
Resp Rate	30-40 per minute	normal for age
I:E ratio[1]	1:2	1 : 2
Setting	PIP[2] causing adequate rise and fall of chest with good breath sounds. In well newborn, this is ~ 15 cm H_2O. If older or lung disease ~ 20-30 cm H_2O.	tidal volume 10-12 ml/kg
PEEP[3]	start at 3-4 cm H_2O	start at 3-4 cm H_2O
FiO_2	5-10% above preintubation FiO_2, adjust to oxygen saturation	

[1] Inspiratory/expiratory ratio, which varies with higher respiratory rate and specific diseases.
[2] Peak inspiratory pressure.
[3] Peak end expiratory pressure.

Analgesia and Sedation

Agent Trade name	Dose (mg/kg)	Route	Onset (min)	Duration (hours)	Comments & Select Properties[1]
alfentanil *Alfenta*	5-20 µg/kg	IV	1-3	0.5	Not approved < 12 y, inject slowly over 3-5 min, chest wall rigidity
chloral hydrate	50-75	PO/PR	10-20	4-8	GI irritant, rare cardiac arrhythmias, possible carcinogen
diazepam *Valium*	0.1 0.2-0.5	IV PR	< 1	1-2	↓respirations, ↓BP
etomidate *Amidate*	0.1-0.4	IV	< 1	< 0.25	Administer over 1 min, causes myoclonus, vomiting
fentanyl *Sublimaze*	1-3 µg/kg	IV	2-3	0.5	↓respirations, ↓BP, bradycardia, rare chest wall rigidity
flumazenil *Romazicon*	0.01- 0.03	IV	< 1	1	reverses benzodiazepines (e.g. lorazepam, midazolam, diazepam)
ketamine *Ketalar*	1-2 4 5-10	IV IM PO	< 1 5 30	0.25 0.5-1.0 1-2	↑BP, ↑intracranial/ocular pressure, rare laryngospasm, co-administer atropine .01 mg/kg to ↓salivation
meperidine *Demerol*	1 1-2	IV IM	< 1 0.25	0.5-1.0 2-3	↓respirations, ↓BP, anticholinergic properties
methohexital *Brevital*	20	PR	15	0.5	↓respirations, ↓BP
midazolam *Versed*	0.10 0.15 0.2-0.3	IV IM PR	2 10-15 10-15	0.5 0.75 1	↓respirations, ↓BP Start IV dose at 0.05-0.10 mg/kg with slow titration to max of 0.4-0.5 mg/kg
morphine	0.1	IV	< 5	3-4	↓respirations, ↓BP
naloxone *Narcan*	0.1	IV, IM, SC	< 1	< 1	Reverses narcotics Erratic absorption SC
nitrous oxide	30%	inhaled	1-2	< 0.1	Patient holds mask to self-titrate
propofol *Diprivan*	0.5-1.0	IV	< 1	< 0.25	Painful injection, contraindicated < 3 years old, PICU, allergy to egg yolk, lecithin, soybean oil, glycerol, EDTA (infusion 25-125 µg/kg/min after bolus)
thiopental *Pentothal*	3-5 5-10	IV PR	< 1 5	0.1-0.5 0.5-1.0	Slow IV at 1 mg/kg q 1-2 min. Causes histamine release, ↓respiration, ↓BP

[1]Caution should be exercised with use of these agents. Only those thoroughly familiar with pediatric airway management, appropriate monitoring, and knowledgeable regarding action and side effect should administer these agents.

Oral Analgesic Agents

Agent	Dose (mg/kg)	Frequency	Concentration / Comments
acetaminophen	15	q4h	80 mg/0.8 ml (dropper) or 160 mg per 5 ml
acetaminophen with codeine	0.5 to 1	q4h	acetaminophen 120 mg + codeine 12 mg per 5 ml (dose in mg/kg based on codeine)
aspirin	10-15	q4h	no elixir available
hydrocodone[1] (*Lortab* elixir)	-	q4-6h	Dose: > 12 years – 10 ml q 4-6 hours Dose: 6 - 12 years – 5 ml q 4-6 hours 2.5 mg hydrocodone/167 APAP/5 ml
Ibuprofen (susp)	5-10	q4-8h	*Children's Motrin or Advil:* 100 mg per 5 ml
meperidine[1]	1-2	q4h	50 mg per 5 ml
naproxen[1]	5-7	q8h	125 mg per 5 ml

[1]only approved for select ages/indications, consult manufacturer's product labeling.

Maximum Dose of Local Anesthetics Without & (With) Epinephrine

lidocaine (*Xylocaine*)[1]	5 mg/kg (*7 mg/kg*)
bupivicaine (*Marcaine, Sensorcaine*) [2]	2.5 mg/kg (*3 mg/kg*)
mepivicaine (*Carbocaine*)	4 mg/kg (*7 mg/kg*)
prilocaine (never use < 6 months old)	5.5 mg/kg (*8.5 mg/kg*)

[1] For IV regional anesthesia (Bier blocks) max lidocaine dose is 3 mg/kg with even less for mini-Bier block. Use preservative free lidocaine without epinephrine for Bier or hematoma blocks.
[2] Due to cardiac toxicity, never use for IV regional anesthesia or hematoma block.

Technique for mini-Bier block – Regional Anesthesia

Indication – fracture reduction below the elbow.
Medication – 0.5% lidocaine without epinephrine, without preservatives

- Insert IV line in dorsum of ipsilateral hand ± contralateral arm for resuscitation.
- Place double pneumatic or 2 single pneumatic tourniquets above elbow.
- Exsanguinate limb by elevation for few min. or by elevation + wrapping arm with Esmarch rubber or Ace elastic bandage in distal to proximal fashion.
- With extremity elevated, inflate proximal cuff 50 mm Hg above systolic BP.
- Remove bandage and lower extremity back to horizontal.
- Tourniquet pressure must be maintained 50 mm Hg > systolic BP throughout.
- Infuse 1.5 mg/kg diluted to total of 10 ml into hand IV over 60-90 seconds.
- Successful block may manifest as blanching skin with erythematous patches.
- As paresthesia/warmth spreads proximally, the lower/distal cuff is inflated to 50 mm Hg above systolic BP followed by deflation of the proximal cuff. The tourniquet pressure is now exerted over an already anesthetized area. Anesthesia is usually complete by 10 minutes with muscle relaxation. Tactile and proprioceptive sensation, with some motor function may be retained.
- Infuse additional 0.5 mg/kg of 0.5% lidocaine if anesthesia poor at 15 minutes.
- Do not exceed maximum dose of 100 mg IV.
- Once adequate anesthesia reached, remove IV and bandage site.
- Leave tourniquet in place at least 15-20 min. & no more than 60-90 min. after infusion. When procedure finished, completely deflate cuff in cycles for 5 sec., then reinflate X 2 minutes. Repeat inflation/deflation (5 sec/2min) several times until capillary refill normal. Observe at least 1 hour before discharge.

Anaphylaxis

Anaphylaxis Treatment

Drug	Dose -mg/kg	Route	Indications
epinephrine	0.01	SC/IM	mild to moderate symptoms
	infusion[1]	IV	airway compromise, severe hypotension administer 0.1 ml/kg (10 µg/kg) of 1:10,000 solution IV over 2 minutes
methylprednisolone	2	IV	moderate/severe symptoms
diphenhydramine	1	IV/IM	moderate/severe symptoms
cimetidine	5	IV/IM	if no resp. symptoms (bronchoconstricts)
glucagon	0.02-0.03 max 1 mg	IV/SC	if patient taking a β-blocker > 20 kg use 1 mg individual dose (max)
albuterol	2.5-5 mg	nebulized	bronchospasm
epinephrine	0.25-0.5 ml	nebulized	Stridor

[1]*Epinephrine infusion:* see page 191. Use caution, as lethal complications can occur.
Bee Sting Remove stinger, rinse, apply ice. 0.005 ml/kg epi locally if not end-organ site.

Apparent Life Threatening Events (ALTE)

Apnea – cessation of breathing for > 20 seconds or shorter cessation associated with bradycardia, pallor, or cyanosis. **ALTE** – apnea associated with color change (cyanosis, gray, or pallor), a loss of muscle tone, and choking or gagging. (formerly known as near SIDS).

Evaluation and Management
- ADMIT all with true ALTE episode
- Immediately apply cardiac monitor, check O₂ saturation and glucose
- Obtain the following on all patients – CBC, electrolytes, ECG, CXR.
- Consider further tests based on history/exam – spinal tap, UA, EEG, barium swallow, cranial CT, nasopharyngeal RSV swab and pertussis, echocardiogram, sleep studies, Holter, video surveillance

Most Common Causes of ALTE Presenting to a Pediatric ED	
Seizure (afebrile)	25%
Gastroesophageal reflux	18%
Febrile seizure	12%
Lower resp. tract infection	9%
Apnea	9%
Pertussis	6%
Choking	5%
Upper resp. tract infection	4%
Cyanotic episode	2%
Gastroenteritis	2%
Asthma, Head Injury, Feeding difficulty, UTI, Vomiting, Startle response,	each
Rigor, Vaccine reaction, Sepsis, Pallor, Apnea alarm, Developmental delay, Subglottic stenosis	< 1% each

The presence of poor tone, abnormal color change, or need for stimulation does not predict those who will go on to have further apneic or bradycardic episodes.

Pediatr Emerg Care 1999; 195; *Clin Pediatr* 1998; 223.

Visit www.bt.cdc.gov for updates/information re: biologic/chemical exposures.
Visit www.orau.gov/reacts/care.htm or Call (615) 576-1004 re: radiation exposure.
CDC Bioterrorism Preparedness and Response Center 1-770-488-7100
General rules. Gown, gloves, & HEPA filter masks protect vs most biological
agents, soap/water remove most biologic agents from skin, hypochlorites (0.1%)
bleach remove most contaminants from objects.
Anthrax – *Incubation* - usually < 1 week ± 2 mo. *Features* – fever, myalgia, cough,
chest pain, dyspnea, shock. Skin - edema, then pruritic macule/papule, ulcer,
painless, depressed eschar, lymphangitis, painful lymphadenopthy, *Diagnosis* –
CXR-wide mediastinum ± effusion, Wright or Gram stain blood, blood cultures,
ELISA for toxin. *Chemoprophylaxis* – (1) ciprofloxacin 10-15 mg/kg PO q 12 h (max
1 g/d) X 60 d OR (2) doxycycline (2a) > 8 years & > 45 kg: 100 mg PO BID X 60
days OR (2b) ≤ 8 years or < 45 kg: 2.2 mg/kg PO BID X 60 d OR (3) amoxicillin 80
mg/kg divided tid X 60 d *if penicillin sensitive*. *Treatment* – inhaled, systemic (all
ages) & cutaneous (if < 2 y). (1) ciprofloxacin IV [see above –if meningitis
possible] **OR** (2) doxycycline 2.2 mg/kg IV q 12 h **PLUS** 1 or 2 of following agents:
clindamycin 30 mg/kg/day (q 6-8 h), rifampin, vancomycin, penicillin, ampicillin,
chloramphenicol, imipenem, or clarithromycin. See page 77-85 for dosing.
Blistering Agents – Mustard gas - severe skin, lung, or eye damage with delayed
blisters up to 12-18 hours. Smell - mustard, onion, or garlic. Skin is red & blisters
form. Airway irritation is prominent early. Treat supportively. **Lewisite** - immediate
burn eyes, nose, & skin (flushed). Treat by decontaminating & using dimercaprol.
Botulinum – *Onset* – 1-5 days. *Features* – afebrile, descending symmetric flaccid
paralysis starts at cranial nerves. Respiratory failure ± in 24 hours. Foodborne.
Diagnosis – nasal swab ELISA. *Treatment* – supportive, trivalent (vs. A,B,C) or
pentavalent (vs. A to E) antitoxin may prevent progression, can give pre-exposure.
Brucellosis –aerosol or food source *Incubation* – 8-14 days. *Features* – fever,
headache, fatigue, colitis, hepatitis, arthritis, lymph nodes, osteomyelitis, epididy-
moorchitis, endocarditis ± recurrence, *Diagnosis* – blood & bone marrow culture, or
serology, *Prophylaxis* – doxycycline [anthrax dose] or ciprofloxacin 15-20 mg/kg X 3
weeks. *Treatment* – (1) doxycycline [anthrax dose] + rifampin [20 mg/kg/day] X 6
weeks OR (2) doxycycline X 6 weeks + streptomycin 30 mg/kg/day IM X 3 weeks.
Cyanide – colorless, inhale > ingest, bitter almond smell. H/A, dyspnea, HTN, ↑
HR then apnea, ↓BP, ↓ HR, seizure, dysrhythmias, cell death. Retinal veins cherry
red. Labs – ↑ anion gap acidosis, venous pO₂ > 40 mm Hg. Treat - Lilly antidote kit
(1) –inhale amyl nitrate 30 sec/min until IV meds ready; (2) Na nitrate (10%) 0.33
ml/kg (10ml/300 mg max) IV. Use less if anemic. May ↓BP, methem-oglobinemia
(goal MetHb ≤ 25%); (3) Na+ thiosulfate (25%) 1.65 ml/kg (12.5 g/50 ml max) IV.
Nerve Agents – (**GF, Sarin, Soman, Tabun, VX**) –inhaled & dermally absorbed
cholinesterase inhibitors (organophosphates). Causes CNS Δ (delirium, confusion,
seizures, resp. depression), muscarinic (SLUDGE: salivate, lacrimate, urinate,
defecation, GI, emesis, & miosis, bronchoconstrict, ↓HR) & nicotinic (muscles
weak, HTN, ↑HR, ± mydriasis). Manage (1) decontaminate (rescuers wear
protection),(2) resp support (3) ↑ dose atropine, (4) pralidoxime (esp. Sarin,
Soman). See page 157 for dose.

Phosgene – smells like newly mowed hay. Inhalation causes irritation to eyes, nose, skin producing tissue damage within minutes of contact. Chest tightness, difficulty breathing, and delayed pulmonary edema occur. Treat supportively.

Plague – *Incubation* 1-10 days. *Features* – bubonic (malaise, fever, purulent lymphadenitis), sepsis, or pneumonic plague. CXR – patchy/consolidated pneumonia. *Diagnosis* – Wright-Giemsa or gram stain, culture of blood, lymph node aspirate or sputum. ELISA and IFA tests *Chemoprophylaxis* (1) Septra – 8-12 mg/kg/d trimethoprim divided bid, OR doxycycline (2a) > 8 years & > 45 kg: 100 mg PO BID X 7 days OR (2b) ≤ 8 years or < 45 kg: 2.2 mg/kg PO BID X 7 d. *Treatment* – (1) gentamicin 2.5 mg/kg IV q 8 h OR (2) streptomycin 30 mg/kg/d (bid) ADD (3) chloramphenical 75-100 mg/kg/day divide q 6 h if meningitis X 14 d.

Q fever – *Coxiella burnetii (rickettsia-like)* *Incubation* 10-40 days, *Features* - fever, ± atypical pneumonia/hilar lymph nodes, hepatitis. *Diagnosis* – ELISA, *Treatment* – ciprofloxacin or doxycycline X 7 days [anthrax dose], macrolides may be effective.

Radiation – *Features* – acute radiation syndrome – 1st prodrome: nausea, vomiting, diarrhea, fatigue X 1-2 days, ± burns (±7-10 days to blister) 2nd symptom free latency (absent if > 1000 rads), 3rd overt symptoms: GI (vomiting, diarrhea, bleed, sepsis), CNS (confusion, edema), Heme (↓WBC [lymphocytes] Hb & platelets ± delayed 2-3 weeks if low dose) *Treatment* – Protective clothes, radiation monitor for medical personnel. Treat trauma, externally decontaminate. Admit if ≥ 200 rads. If no symptoms 1st 24 h, exposure is < 75 rads. CBC& diff. q 6-8 hours. Reverse isolation, anti-emetics, colony stimulation factor, stem cell, platelet & Hb transfusion, tissue & blood typing (family/marrow transplant). Prophylactic antibiotics, antivirals, anti-fungals prn. Radioactive fallout from radioactive iodine (e.g. nuclear reactor) causes exposure via inhalation, or ingestion (e.g cow's milk) resulting in cancer (esp. thyroid). Depending on thyroid exposure in rads, potassium iodide (KI) is recommended by CDC.

Population	Predicted thyroid exposure	Daily KI dose
Adults over 40 years	> 500 rad	130 mg
Adults > 18 to 40 years	≥ 10	130 mg
Pregnancy or lactating	≥ 5	130 mg
> 12 to 18 years (if ≥ 70 kg, treat as adult)	≥ 5	65 mg
> 3 to 12 years	≥ 5	65 mg
> 1 mo to 3 years (dilute in milk, formula, H$_2$0)	≥ 5	32 mg
0-1 months	≥ 5	16 mg

Do not give if known iodine sensitive, dermatitis herpetiformis, or hypocomplement-emic vasculitis & use cautiously if thyroid disease. KI protects only thyroid gland from radioiodines, offers no protection from external radiation, does not protect from effect of exposure to other radioactive materials. KI lasts 24 h, use daily until no risk
www.fda.gov/cder/guidance/index.htm

Ricin – type II ribosome inactivation from castor beans/seeds. *Onset* – 4-8 h after inhaled, *Features* – ingestion - vomiting, diarrhea, GI necrosis, hepatitis; inhalation – pulm necrosis, shock. *Diagnosis* – ELISA, *Treat*– supportive, GI decontamination

Smallpox – orthopox virus. *Incubation* – 7-17 days. *Features* – fever, headache, backache. Maculopapular rash face > mouth/pharynx, mucosa & arms/legs, palms, soles (*Varicella* causes rash on trunk > other areas, at different stages, & *no palm/sole involvement*). 1-2 days rash is vesicular, then pustular. Round/tense pustules deeply embedded with crusting on 8th day. All lesions occur/evolve at same rate. *Diagnosis* - Vesicle/pustule fluid or scabs can be examined by electron microscope. *Treatment* – isolate and provide support. *Cidofovir* is effective in vitro.

Staphylococcal enterotoxin B –inhaled or ingested. *Onset* – 3-12 hours *Features* – sudden fever (lasts up to 5 days), headache, chills, dyspnea, vomiting, diarrhea (if swallowed aerosol), with cough up to 4 weeks. CXR - normal, although ARDS can develop. *Diagnosis* – clinically differentiated by abrupt onset in large numbers of exposed presenting at same time, normal CXR, & non-progression. Toxin is difficult to identify. ELISA nasal swabs in 1st 24 h may be +. *Treatment* - supportive

Trichothecene Mycotoxins – fungal toxins (e.g. yellow rain) inhibit protein & DNA synthesis, and destroy cells. *Onset* – minutes to hours. *Features* -Skin damage (blisters). Ingestion: vomiting, bloody diarrhea, and GI bleed. Inhalation: acute eye pain/red, tears, bloody rhinorrhea, hemoptysis + skin findings, ARDS, ↓ BP, bone marrow depression and sepsis. *Diagnosis* – gas liquid chromatography blood, urine, stool, lung washings. *Treatment* – supportive, ascorbic acid, dexamethasone, GI decontamination/lavage, skin (soap/water), eye (saline irrigation).

Tularemia – *Francisella tularensis* (gram negative bacillus). *Incubation* – 2-10 days. *Features* –glandular (nodes without ulcer), ulceroglandular (indurated, punched out ulcers with lymphadenitis, draining nodes with 10-30% pneumonic), pneumonic (atypical fulminant effusion) or septic form (80% have pneumonia). *Diagnosis* – serology (ELISA), culture sputum, fasting gastric aspirate, pharyngeal washings. *Chemoprophylaxis* – same as anthrax dose X 14 days. *Treat* – (1) gentamicin 2.5 mg/kg q 8h X 10-14 days OR (2) spectinomycin.

Viral Encephalitides – (Venezuelan/VEE, eastern/EEE & western equine/WEE) highly infectious by aerosol. *Incubation* – VEE 2-6 days, EEE/WEE 7-14 days. *Features* – fever, headache, myalgias. VEE will cause symptoms in almost all infected, only 0.5-4 % develop neurologic involvement. EEE will kill 50-75%. *Diagnosis* – CSF - pleocytosis, acutely IgM antibodies, ELISA, & hemagglutination-inhibiting antibodies are positive by second week. *Treatment* – supportive care.

Viral Hemorrhagic fevers –due to a variety of RNA viruses (e.g. Marburg, Ebola). *Incubation* - 4-21 days. *Features* – fever, myalgias, prostration, early conjunctival injection, mild hypotension, flushing, petechial hemorrhages. Later DIC picture with hepatitis, renal failure and CV collapse. *Diagnosis* – ELISA, or reverse transcriptase polymerase chain reaction. *Treatment* –Ribavirin and convalescent plasma containing neutralizing antibodies may be useful for specific strains.

Yellow Fever – Flavovirus. *Incubation* – 3-6 days. *Features* – fever, jaundice, proteinuria, hemorrhage. *Prophylaxis* – vaccine available. *Treatment* – supportive.

Burns and Burn Therapy

Fluid resuscitation in burn victims

Parkland formula	• Lactated ringers 4 ml/kg/% burn BSA[1] in 1st 24 h + maintenance fluid, with ½ over 1st 8 hours, and ½ over subsequent 16 h
Alternatives (See page 51 for maintenance fluid rate)	• *Amended Parkland formula:* for ED stays < 8 hours. IV rate over maintenance[2] (ml/h) = [weight(kg) X burn BSA%] ÷ 4 • *Carvajal's formula:* Carvajal' sol'n 5,000 ml/m² of burn + maintenance 2000 ml/m² in 1st 24h, ½ in 1st 8h + ½ over next 16h. • *Monafo* (250 mEq Na/L), *Slater* (LR + 75 ml/kg/day FFP), *Warden* (LR + 50 meq NaHCO₃/L) to keep UO 30-50 ml/h (0.5-1 kg/kg/h)

[1]BSA = body surface area.

Estimation of Burn Surface Area

Age in Years	<1	1	5	10	15
head	19%	17%	13%	11%	9%
neck	2	2	2	2	2
half of trunk(ant or post)	13	13	13	13	13
one buttock	2.5	2.5	2.5	2.5	2.5
genitalia	1	1	1	1	1
upper (3) or lower (4) arm	3-4	3-4	3-4	3-4	3-4
one hand (2.5) or foot (3.5)	2.5-3.5	2.5-3.5	2.5-3.5	2.5-3.5	2.5-3.5
one thigh	5	6.5	8.5	9	9.5
one leg (below knee)	5	5	5.5	6	6.5

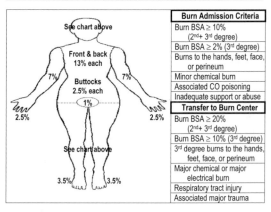

Burn Admission Criteria
Burn BSA ≥ 10% (2nd+ 3rd degree)
Burn BSA ≥ 2% (3rd degree)
Burns to the hands, feet, face, or perineum
Minor chemical burn
Associated CO poisoning
Inadequate support or abuse

Transfer to Burn Center
Burn BSA ≥ 20% (2nd+ 3rd degree)
Burn BSA ≥ 10% (3rd degree)
3rd degree burns to the hands, feet, face, or perineum
Major chemical or major electrical burn
Respiratory tract injury
Associated major trauma

Cardiology – Arrhythmias & ECG evaluation

Normal ECG Values

Age	P-R interval[a]	QRS interval[a]	QRS axis (mean)	QTc[b]
0-7 days	0.08-0.12	0.04-0.08	80-160 (125)	0.34-0.54
1-4 weeks	0.08-0.12	0.04-0.07	60-160 (110)	0.30-0.50
1-3 months	0.08-0.12	0.04-0.08	40-120 (80)	0.32-0.47
3-6 months	0.08-0.12	0.04-0.08	20-80 (65)	0.35-0.46
6-12 months	0.09-0.13	0.04-0.08	0-100 (65)	0.31-0.49
1-3 years	0.10-0.14	0.04-0.08	20-100 (55)	0.34-0.49
3-8 years	0.11-0.16	0.05-0.09	40-80 (60)	< 0.45
8-16 years	0.12-0.17	0.05-0.09	20-80 (60)	< 0.45

[a] seconds [b] QTc = QT interval / (square root of RR interval)

ECG Diagnosis of Chamber Enlargement (Hypertrophy)

Right ventricular hypertrophy/RVH
- R in V1 > 20 mm (> 25 mm < 1 mo)
- S in V6 > 6 mm (> 12 mm < 1 mo)
- Upright T in V3R, R in V1 after 5 day
- QR pattern in V3R, V1

Left ventricular hypertrophy/LVH
- R in V6 > 25 mm (> 21 mm < 1 yr)
- S in V1 > 30 mm (> 20 mm < 1 yr)
- R in V6 + S in V1 > 60 mm (use V5 if R in V5 > R in V6)
- Abnormal R/S ratio
- S in V1 > 2 X R in V5

Biventricular hypertrophy
- RVH and (S in V1 or R in V6) exceeding mean for age
- LVH and (R in V1 or S in V6) exceeding mean for age

Right atrial hypertrophy
- peak P value > 3 mm (< 6 months), > 2.5 mm (≥ 6 months)

Left atrial hypertrophy
- P in II > 0.09 seconds
- P in V1 with late negative deflection > 0.04 seconds and > 1 mm deep

ECG Findings in Medical Disorders

Disorder	Typical ECG Findings (not necessarily most common)
Calcium	*Hyper* - short QT, AV block, ↓ HR, *Hypo* - long QT, ↑ HR
CNS bleed	Diffuse deep T inversion, prominent U, QT > 60% of normal
Digoxin effect	Downward curve of ST segment, flat/inverted T's, short QT
Drug toxicity	See specific drugs and effects pages 140-160
Hyperkalemia	Peaked T's, then flat P's, wide QRS and QT, sine wave
Hypokalemia	Flat T waves, U waves, ST depression
Thyroid	*Hypo* - ↓ HR, ↓ voltage, ST ↓, flat/↓ T waves; *Hyper* - ↑HR
Kawasaki disease	Prolonged P-R, nonspecific ST-T changes,
Lyme disease	AV block, pericarditis, intraventricular conduction delays
Myocarditis	Diffuse nonspecific ST-T △, AV block, ventricular ectopy
Pericarditis	Flat/concave ST ↑, PR segment depression, ↓ voltage

Arrhythmias

Bradycardia

- Assess ABC's
- Secure airway
- Administer 100% oxygen
- Assess vital signs
- Start IV or intraosseous line

↓

NO ← Severe cardiopulmonary compromise?
(poor perfusion, ↓BP, or respiratory difficulty) → **YES**

↓

• Observe • Support ABC's • Consider transfer to advanced life support facility	During CPR Attempt/verify/check • Tracheal intubation & vascular access • Electrode, paddle, pacer & contacts Administer • Epinephrine q 3-5 min ± epinephrine or dopamine infusion • Identify/treat head injury, hypothermia hypoxia, heart block, toxin, transplant	Chest compressions if despite O₂, ventilation • HR < 60 in infant or child and poor systemic perfusion

The middle and right columns are linked by ← →

↓ (right column)

Epinephrine
- IV/IV – 0.01 mg/kg (1:10,000 – 0.1 ml/kg)
- Tracheal – 0.1 mg/kg (1:1000 – 0.1 ml/kg)
- Repeat q 3-5 min

↓

Atropine 0.02 mg/kg (min dose 0.1 mg). May repeat once. Give 1st if bradycardia due to vagal tone or primary AV block

↓

If pulseless arrest develops, See Pulseless Arrest Algorithm (page 9) ←
- Consider external or esophageal pacing
- Consider digoxin Fab fragments if digoxin toxicity
- Consider glucagon if toxicity from β-blockers or calcium channel blockers

Differentiation of Sinus Tachycardia from Supraventricular Tachycardia

	Sinus Tachycardia	Supraventricular Tachycardia
History	Volume loss (dehydration, bleed), Drugs, Other stressor	Often vague & nondescript, if prolonged - CHF or shock
Heart rate < 1 year	< 220	≥220
Heart rate > 1 year	< 180-200	> 180-200
QRS width	Narrow for age	Narrow in 90%
P waves	Upright leads I, aVF	Rare, neg. in II, III, aVF
HR & R-R variability	Beat-beat (R-R varies), responds to stimulation	No variability, no response to stimulation
HR changes	Slow increase or decrease	Abrupt onset and termination

Stable Tachycardia Management

Assess/support ABCs, O₂, Attach monitor & defibrillator, Evaluate ECG if possible, Start IV

Is QRS wide for age (~ ≤ or > 0.08 seconds)? See page 21 for age based normal QRS duration

Narrow QRS AND Supraventricular Tachycardia See chart above (SVT vs. ST)	Wide Complex - Probable Ventricular Tachycardia

During evaluation provide O₂, consider cardiology consult, prepare cardioversion 0.5 to 1.0 J/kg and sedation. **Identify/treat** possible causes: ↓ O₂, ↓ volume, ↑Temp., ↓ or ↑ K⁺, Metabolic disorders, Tamponade, Tension Pneumothorax, Toxins/Drugs, Pain, & Thromboembolism

Consider vagal maneuvers

Adenosine 0.1 mg/kg (max 6 mg), repeat at 0.2 mg/kg (max 12mg), IV bolus, 5 ml NS flush

Consult pediatric cardiologist Attempt cardioversion at 0.5 to 1.0 J/kg, with ↑ to 2 J/kg Sedate prior to cardioversion	Consider medications¹ Amiodarone 5 mg/kg IV over 20 to 60 minutes OR Procainamide 15 mg/kg IV over 30 to 60 minutes OR Lidocaine 1 mg/kg IV

¹Consider MgSO₄ 25 mg/kg IV over 15 min if torsades   *Circulation* 2000; 102: I-315

Wide Supraventricular Tachycardia (Aberrancy) vs. Ventricular Tachycardia[1]

	Supraventricular Tachycardia	Ventricular Tachycardia
History	WPW in up to 30% in infancy[2]	70% structural cardiac dz.
Symptoms & BP	Not a useful differentiator	Not a useful differentiator
Heart rate	> 220 infant, > 180 child	> 120
P waves	Retrograde P waves possible	Dissociation of P & QRS
Other features	Features found useful in differentiating adult VT (*absence of RS in all precordial leads, QRS concordance in precordial leads, QRS ≥ 0.12-0.14 ms* vs SVT (*triphasic QRS with RBBB in V1 or V6*) have not been studied in children	

[1]During management, generally assume wide complex tachy is ventricular tachycardia.
[2]Ebstein's anomaly esp. associated with WPW in 10-30%

Unstable Tachycardia Management[1]

Assess/support ABCs, O₂, Attach monitor & defibrillator, Evaluate ECG if possible, Start IV

Is QRS wide for age (~ ≤ or > 0.08 seconds)?
See page 21 for age-based normal QRS duration

Narrow QRS AND Supraventricular Tachycardia
See chart page 23 (SVT vs. ST)

Wide Complex - Probable Ventricular Tachycardia

During evaluation provide O₂, consider cardiology consult, prepare cardioversion 0.5 to 1.0 J/kg and sedation (if therapy not delayed)
Identify/treat causes: ↓ O₂, ↓ volume, ↑Temp., ↓ or ↑ K⁺, Metabolic disorders, Tamponade, Tension Pneumothorax, Toxins/Drugs, Pain, & Thromboembolism

Consider vagal maneuvers
without delay

Immediate cardioversion
0.5 to 1.0 J/kg (consider sedation)
Increase to 2 J/kg if ineffective
OR
Adenosine 0.1 mg/kg (max 6 mg), repeat at 0.2 mg/kg (max 12mg), IV bolus, 5 ml NS flush

Immediate cardioversion
0.5 to 1.0 J/kg (consider sedation)
Increase to 2 J/kg if ineffective

Consider medications
Amiodarone 5 mg/kg IV over 20 to 60 minutes **OR**
Procainamide 15 mg/kg IV over 30 to 60 minutes **OR**
Lidocaine 1 mg/kg IV

[1]See page 9 for pulseless VF/VT, PEA management   *Circulation 2000; 102: I-316*

Other Rhythm/ECG disturbances

Atrial flutter - atrial rate of 250-350 beats/minute with variable but regular ventricular rate depending on degree of AV block. 93% have structural heart disease often post-surgical. Treat if unstable with synchronized cardioversion – initially use 0.5 J/kg doubling to 1 J/kg, then 2 J/kg if needed. Digoxin, procainamide, & amiodarone are used in hemodynamically stable patients.

Atrial Fibrillation - atrial rate of > 300-600 with irregularly irregular ventricular rates often > 100-150 beats/minute. As with Aflutter, most infants have structural heart disease, & management of unstable patients requires synchronized cardioversion. If stable, anticoagulation is usually required before converting rhythm.

Prolonged QT interval - (1) inherited form may be associated with deafness, or (2) acquired due to class I antiarrhythmics (e.g., quinidine, procainamide), amiodarone, phenothiazines, lithium, cyclic antidepressants, ↓K+, ↓Ca+2, ↓Mg+2, myocarditis, liver disease, weight loss. Children with prolonged QTc may present with syncope or seizures. Treat by correcting disorder or discontinuing drug. QTc = QT interval / (square root of RR interval). See page 21 for age-based normal QTc intervals.

Torsade de pointes –polymorphic VT with morphology swinging from negative to positive direction in 1 lead. Etiology: see ↑ QT above. Treat: fix underlying disease, $MgSO_4$ 25 mg/kg slow IV, overdrive pacing, isoproterenol, lidocaine, phenytoin.

Select Anti-Arrhythmic Agents

Adenosine/_Adenocard_ – endogenous purine nucleoside used to treat SVT.
<u>Dose:</u> 0.1 mg/kg IV push (max 6 mg), may double and repeat at 0.2 mg/kg (max 12 mg) every 1-2 minutes to a maximum of 0.3 mg/kg (max 12 mg) or SVT termination.
<u>Contraindications</u> – sick sinus syndrome, 2nd or 3rd degree AV block, current use of digoxin and verapamil (may precipitate Vfib), asthma (may precipitate bronchospasm esp. if using theophylline), carbemazepine/_Tegretol_ use (may increase degree of heart block), de-innervated heart (post-transplant)
<u>Side effects</u> – flushing, palpitations, chest pain, bradycardia, heart block, headache, dyspnea, bronchoconstriction in asthmatics

Amiodarone/_Cordarone_ – Class III antiarrhythmic with adrenergic stimulation inhibition, ↑ action potential/refractory period, ↓ AV conduction/sinus node function used for ventricular fibrillation, ventricular tachycardia, SVT, Atrial fib/flutter.
<u>Dose:</u> (pulseless VF/VT) 5 mg/kg rapid IV or IO bolus (max 300 mg). (VT/SVT with pulse) 5 mg/kg IV or IO over 20-60 minutes (max 150 mg). May repeat up to maximum dose of 15 mg/kg/day. IV maintenance dose 5 micrograms/kg/minute (max 15 micrograms/kg/min)
<u>Contraindications</u> – sinus node disease, marked bradycardia, $2^{nd}/3^{rd}$ AV block
<u>Side Effects</u> – ↓ HR resistant to atropine (may need isoproterenol or pacer), ↓ BP, cardiac arrest, torsades de pointes (↑ QT), ARDS/pneumonitis, hepatitis

Select Anti-Arrhythmics – continued

Digoxin/Lanoxin – cardiac glycoside with inotropic and AV blocking effects.

Age	Total digitalizing dose	Maintenance(IV) daily dose
premature neonate	15- 25 µg/kg	4-6 µg/kg
term neonate	20-30 µg/kg	5-8 µg/kg
1-24 months	30-50 µg/kg	7.5-12 µg/kg
2-5 years	25-35 µg/kg	6-9 µg/kg
5-10 years	15-30 µg/kg (max 1.5 mg)	4-8µg/kg

Total digitalizing dose (TDD) is given over 16-24 hours: ½ of dose initially IV, followed by ¼ dose at both 8 and 16 hours. Oral doses are 20% greater, with maintenance dose 12.5% of TDD q12h starting 12h after TDD complete.
<u>Contraindications</u> – ventricular dysrhythmias. In patients receiving digoxin, cardioversion or calcium infusion can precipitate ventricular fibrillation.
<u>Side effects</u> – atrial and supraventricular arrhythmias with or without block, bradycardia, vomiting, diarrhea, headache, confusion.
Esmolol/Brevibloc – β1 selective blocker with short half life (2 minutes).
<u>Dose</u> – 100-500 micrograms/kg IV over 5 minutes with initial maintenance infusion of 50 micrograms/kg/minute. May increase infusion 50 micrograms/kg/min every 5 minutes to maximum of 200 micrograms/kg/min (0.2 mg/kg/min).
<u>Contraindications</u> – sinus bradycardia, or heart block, CHF, cardiogenic shock.
<u>Side effects</u> – hypotension, bradycardia, confusion, vomiting, bronchoconstriction.
Lidocaine – Class IB antiarrhythmic.
<u>Dose</u> – 1 mg/kg IV/IO or 2-10 mg/kg ET. 2nd bolus of 0.5 – 1.0 mg/kg IV/IO (2-10 X higher for ET) if needed. Infusion - 20-50 micrograms/kg/minute.
<u>Contraindications</u> –amide anesthetic allergy, AV, SA, interventricular heart block
<u>Side effects</u> – ↓BP/HR, altered LOC, seizure, vomiting, respiratory depression
Procainimide – Class IA antiarrhythmic with anticholinergic/anesthetic effects
<u>Dose</u> – 15 mg/kg IV over ≥ 30 minutes. Infusion - 20-80 micrograms/kg/min.
<u>Contraindications</u> – 2nd/3rd degree heart block, torsade de pointes, QT prolongation, myasthenia gravis, lupus, hypersensitivity to procaine
<u>Side effects</u> – ↓BP, ↑ or ↓ HR, QT/QRS widening, confusion, vomiting, neutropenia, thrombocytopenia, anemia, ↑ LFTs, lupus-like syndrome
Verapamil – calcium channel blocker with negative inotropic & chronotropic effect
<u>Dose</u>–0.1 mg/kg IV (max 5 mg). Repeat 0.2 mg/kg (max 10mg) in 30 min if no effect
<u>Contraindications</u> – **NEVER** use < 1 year & exercise caution using 1-8 years due to myocardial depression. Other contraindications sinus bradycardia, heart block, shock ventricular tachycardia, wide complex SVT/Afib/Aflutter due to bypass tract.
<u>Side effects</u> – ↓BP/HR, heart block, CHF, seizures, respiratory insufficiency in muscular dystrophy, ↑ LFTs, GI upset, constipation

Chest Pain

Cardiac Causes of Chest Pain in Children

• Ischemia from arteritis (Kawasaki's), coronary anomalies, HTN, $\downarrow O_2$ • Structural anomalies (e.g. aortic stenosis), pulmonic stenosis, idiopathic subaortic stenosis (IHSS)	• Arrhythmias ($\downarrow$ or $\uparrow$HR) • $\downarrow$ BP with$\downarrow$ coronary perfusion • Infectious or inflammatory disease (e.g. pericarditis, myocarditis, endocarditis)

Chest Pain Etiologies Presenting to a Pediatric Emergency Department	Musculoskeletal	25%	Psychogenic	9%
	Respiratory	21%	Trauma	5%
	Idiopathic	21%	GI	4%
	Miscellaneous	11%	Cardiac	4%

Pediatrics 1988; 82: 319

Congenital Heart Disease

Most Common Congenital Defects Diagnosed at Different Ages[1]

0-6 Days		7-13 Days		14-28 Days	
D-Transposition of great arteries	19%	Coarctation-aorta	16%	VSD	16%
Hypoplastic LH	14%	VSD	14%	Coarctation-aorta	12%
Tetrology of Fallot	8%	Hypoplastic LH	8%	Tetrology of Fallot	7%
Coarctation–aorta	7%	D-Transposition of great arteries	7%	D-Transposition of great arteries	7%
VSD	3%	Tetrology of Fallot	7%	Patent ductus	5%
Other defects	49%	Other defects	48%	Other defects	53%

[1]LH – left heart, VSD – ventricular septal defect   *Clin Perinatology* 2001; 28: 91.

Hyperoxia Test for Diagnosing Cyanotic Congenital Heart Disease[4]

Specific Disorders[1]	PaO$_2$ (%sat) FiO$_2$ 21%	PaO$_2$ (%sat)[2] FiO$_2$ 100%	PaCO$_2$
No disease	> 70 (>95%)	> 300 (100%)	35
Lung or neurologic disease	> 50 (85%)	> 150 (100%)	50
D-TGA ± VSD, Tricuspid atresia+ PS or atresia, critical PS, Tetralogy of Fallot	< 40 (< 75%)	< 50 (< 85%)	35
Truncus arteriosus, TAPV, Hypoplastic left heart, Single ventricle	40-60 (75-93%)	< 150 (<100%)	35
Persistent pulm. HTN of newborn, LV outflow tract obstruct (AA hypoplasia, interrupted AA, critical coarctation, AS)	Pre 70 (95)[3] Post < 40 (< 75)	Variable	35-50
D-TGA + (coarctation of aorta or interrupted aortic arch) or + pulmonary AS	Pre <40 (<75) Post >50 (<90)	Variable	35-50

[1] TGA – transposition of great arteries, PS – pulmonary stenosis, TAPV – total anomalous pulmonary venous return, HTN – hypertension, AA – aortic arch, AS – aortic stenosis
[2] Perform post ABG after 10 min of 100% O_2, [3]Defect is (pre)ductal or (post)ductal
[4] A neonate who fails a hyperoxia test is likely to have ductal dependent systemic or pulmonary blood flow and should receive PGE$_1$ *Clin Perinatology* 2001; 28: 91.

Chest Radiography in Acyanotic Congenital Heart Disease	
Normal pulm. flow	PS, MS or MR, AS, coarctation of the aorta
↑ Pulmonary flow	ASD, VSD, PDA, left to right shunts with pulm HTN, AV canal

Chest Radiography in Cyanotic Congenital Heart Disease	
↓ Pulmonary flow	Severe PS, pulm. atresia, Tetralogy of Fallot (normal/boot shaped heart), TGA with PS, Tricuspid atresia, Ebstein's anomaly (massive heart), Eisenmenger's complex
↑ Pulmonary flow	TAPVR (Snowman sign – late finding, supracardiac venous return via dilated right & left superior vena cava), Hypoplastic LH, TGA (egg shaped heart tilted on its side with a narrow mediastinum "egg on a string") ± VSD, Truncus arteriosus

Acyanotic Heart Disease

Cardiac lesions with flow of blood from high pressure left to right side of the heart via a defect that can cause varying degrees of CHF depending on lesion.

Examples – (1) *atrial septal defect* – often asymptomatic until adulthood & can cause RAE and SVTs. (2) *ventricular septal defects* (VSD) if small may cause loud holosystolic murmur at left sternal border. If moderate, CHF may develop after first few weeks of life as normal newborn pulmonary resistance drops, decreasing RV pressures, and increasing the left to right shunt. RVH > LVH ± LAE may be evident on ECG. (3) *patent ductus arteriosus*. Early systolic/diastolic murmur at 2nd, 3rd left IC space – later becomes machinery type murmur that radiates to the back. Progressive CHF may develop while ECG may show LVH if PDA is large.

Acute Management of CHF – Elevate head of bed, O_2 (caution – O_2 causes↓ pulmonary vasc. resistance & ↑ systemic vasc. resistance, potentially ↑ left to right shunt. In this instance, the goal for O_2 saturation is~ 85%) furosemide (*Lasix*) 1.0 mg/kg IV, morphine 0.05 mg/kg IV, dopamine/dobutamine if shock, vasodilator if ↑BP or vasoconstriction (e.g. nitroprusside), treat underlying cause (transfuse if anemia, antiarrhythmic if SVT, PGE_1 [dose page 191] if ductal dependent lesion - hypoplastic left heart, severe coarctation, interrupted aortic arch, TGA)

Cyanotic Heart Disease with Decreased Pulmonary Flow

Obstruction of flow at the right side of the heart so there is less flow to the lungs Example – (1) *Tetralogy of Fallot* – VSD, right ventricle outflow obstruction, RVH, overriding aorta – ECG may show RVH, RAD. Acute shunting leads to ↑RR, ↑ cyanosis, ↓ murmur, stroke or death. Precipitants: crying, defecating, exercise, ↓ systemic vascular resistance (SVR), ↓ LV pressure, and RV outflow spasm.

Acute Management of hypercyanotic "Tet Spell" – O_2, knee chest position (↓venous return), morphine 0.1 mg/kg IV (↓outflow spasm), NS 20 ml/kg IV (↑SVR),$NaHCO_3$, phenylephrine – 0.1-0.5 µg/kg/min IV (goal = ↑SVR 20%), Prostaglandin E1 (dosing page 191) ± propranolol 0.01 – 0.25 mg/kg slow IV (outflow spasm) [may substitute esmolol] – Use extreme caution. β blockers dramatically ↓BP/HR in neonates.

Cyanotic Heart Disease with Increased Pulmonary Flow

<u>Example</u> – (1) *Transposition of great arteries* – aorta rises from the right ventricle and pulmonary artery from the left ventricle. The only mixing of blood is via foramen ovale, patent ductus arteriosus ± VSD. Patients are cyanotic with congestive heart failure. CXR ± cardiomegaly (egg on a string appearance).
(2) *Total anomalous pulmonary venous return* – all blood (systemic and pulmonary) returns to right atrium. ASD or patent foramen ovale must be present. CXR shows cardiomegaly and increased pulmonary vascular flow. Snowman sign
<u>Acute Management</u> – Treat as CHF, Prostaglandin E1 (dosing page 191)

Left Ventricular Outflow Obstruction

Most common disorders presenting in ≤ 28 day old are hypoplastic left heart (51%), coarctation (34%) and interrupted aortic arch (13%). *Pediatr Emerg Care* 1998; 236.
<u>Examples</u> – (1) hypoplastic left heart – may present early in life with shock ± CHF. Those presenting in first 28 days of life must be differentiated from newborn sepsis. Those with obstructive left heart disease more frequently manifest respiratory distress (87 vs 55%), cardiomegaly (85 vs 5%), murmur (53 vs 5%), ↓ lower ext. pulses (70 vs 11%), ↓ upper extremity pulses (32 vs 3%) and less frequently have irritability (11 vs 55%) and fever (2% vs 53%) compared to newborn with sepsis. Treat with PGE$_1$ (page 191) and early surgical repair. (2) coarctation of the aorta – may present with CHF/cyanosis (preductal), asymptomatic murmur (post ductal), or arterial HTN (↑ BP upper extremities and ↓lower extremities) with weakness/pain lower extremities (3) interrupted aortic arch – may present similar to coarctation. As with coarctation, PGE$_1$ (page 191) is indicated for acute symptoms.

Lesions with ductal dependent Systemic(S) or Pulmonary (P) Flow[1]

Tetralogy of Fallot (P), Ebstein's anomaly (P) Critical PS (P), Tricuspid atresia (P), Pulmonic valve atresia (P)	Hypoplastic left heart (S), Interrupted aortic arch (S), Critical coarctation (S), Critical AS, Tricuspid atresia + TGA (S)

[1]These are mostly disorders with failed hyperoxia test or with shock in the 1st 3 weeks of life. Each may respond to PGE$_1$ (page 191).

Murmurs

Physiologic Murmurs[1]

Murmur	Age	Location	Timing	Cause
Still's	3-6 y	apex	systole	turbulent LV outflow
pulm ejection	8-14 y	2nd left ICS	systole	RV outflow tract turbulence
supraclavicular	4-14 y	above clavicle	systole	brachiocephalic branching
venous hum[2]	3-6 y	base of neck	entire	venous return
straight back pectus	all	apex	systole	RV filling with inspiration
hemic exertion	all	apex, left ICS	systole	rapid LV ejection
neonatal pulm ej	<6 mo	right 2nd ICS	systole	underdeveloped pulm arteries

[1] LV=left ventricle, RV=right ventricle, ICS=intercostal space. Most physiologic murmurs are systolic and are louder with increased cardiac output.
[2] Venous hums decrease with supine position, turning head, and expiration.

Murmurs continued

<u>Murmur evaluation</u>: Murmurs should be of extra concern if the patient has congenital heart disease, failure to thrive, frequent infections, asthma, chest pain, or syncope. Congenital heart disease is suggested if *one* major or *two* minor criteria:

- *Major*: grade ≥ 3, pansystolic, late systolic, diastolic, CHF, cyanosis.
- *Minor*: grade < 3, systolic, or abnormal CXR, ECG, BP, or S_2 heart sound.

Syncope

Syncope Etiologies Presenting to a Pediatric Emergency Department	Vasovagal	50%	Head trauma	5%
	Orthostasis	20%	Migraine	5%
	Atypical seizure	7%	Miscellaneous	13%

Pediatr Emerg Care 1989; 5:80-82

Features Associated with Life Threatening Cause of Syncope

• Family history of cardiomyopathy or sudden death (IHSS, prolonged QT)	• Abnormal ECG
	• Recurrent syncope
• Syncope during exercise or while supine (IHSS, aortic+ pulmonic stenosis, pulmonary hypertension)	• Fall directly onto face (rapid onset)
	• Congenital heart disease
	• Drugs with cardiac effects
• Syncope with chest pain (IHSS, ischemia aortic stenosis)	• Marfanoid appearance or collagen vascular disease in family

American Heart Association/American College of Cardiology Indications for Holter Monitoring in Children.

Class I	• Syncope, near syncope or dizziness if recognized heart disease, previous arrhythmia, pacemaker, or if associated with exertion
	• Evaluation of hypertrophic/dilated cardiomyopathy, long QT
	• Palpitation if prior congenital heart disease (CHD) surgery with residual hemodynamic abnormality.
	• Evaluation of antiarrhythmic drugs during rapid somatic growth
	• Asymptomatic congenital complete AV block, nonpaced
Class IIa	• Syncope, near syncope, sustained palpitation without explanation
	• Evaluate rhythm after starting antiarrhythmic (esp. if proarrhythmic)
	• After transient AV block associated with heart surgery/ablation
	• Evaluate rate responsiveness or physiology pacing function in symptomatic patients
Class IIb	• Asymptomatic prior CHD surgery with residual hemodynamic abnormalities, or significant incidence late postop arrhythmias
	• < 3 yo, prior tachyarrhythmia to look for unrecognized arrhythmia
	• Suspected incessant atrial tachycardia
	• Complex ventricular ectopy on ECG or exercise test
Class III	• Syncope with non cardiac cause,
	• Chest pain with no evidence heart disease
	• Routine athletic clearance, brief palpitation without heart disease
	• Asymptomatic Wolff-Parkinson-White syndrome

I–beneficial, IIa–favors efficacy, IIb–possible efficacy, III – not useful   *JACC 1999; 34: 938.*

Rash Patterns & Etiology

Acneiform	Acne vulgaris, drugs (steroid, Li, INH), Cushing's, chloracne,
Acrodermatitis (extremity)	Papular acrodermatitis, smallpox, atopic dermatitis (infantile), tinea pedis, dyshidrotic eczema, post-strep desquamation, Rocky Mountain spotted fever, drug rash
Clothing-covered	Contact dermatitis, miliaria, psoriasis (summer), folliculitis
Flexural creases	Atopic dermatitis (childhood), infantile seborrheic dermatitis, intertrigo, candidiasis,tinea crurus, icthysosis,inverse psoriasis
Linear Christmas tree distribution	Pityriasis rosea, secondary syphilis, drug reaction, guttate psoriasis, atopic dermatitis
Sun-Exposed	Phototoxic drug rash, photocontact dermatitis, lupus, viral exanthem, porphyria, xeroderma pigmentosum

Vesiculobullous, petechial/purpuric, eczematous, papulosquamous rashes see pg 33-34

Newborn Rashes

Transient benign vascular phenomena (1) *acrocyanosis* - blue, purple discoloration due to cold (2) *cutis marmorata* - reticulated cyanosis/marbling of skin symmetrically involving the trunk and extremities, (3) *harlequin color change* - infant lies horizontally, dependent half becomes bright red in contrast to pale upper half. *Benign pustular dermatoses* in neonates (1) *erythema toxicum neonatorum* - up to 70% of newborns, begins on 2nd/3rd day, lasting up to 3 weeks. 2-3 mm red blotchy macules & papules evolve to pustules with red base. (2) *Transient neonatal pustular melanosis* - 4% of neonates, and is more common in black males. 2-5 mm pustules on a non-erythematous base are present at birth and found on the chin, neck, upper trunk, abdomen and thighs. (3) *Acropustulosis of infancy* - a chronic recurrent pustular eruption on palms/soles, ± scalp, trunk, and extremities. Episodes last 1-3 weeks and can recur until age 3. During flare-ups, infants are fussy, and pruritis is severe. Sterile intradermal pustules occur. Topical steroids relieve symptoms. (4) *Sebaceous gland hyperplasia* due to androgens is common on nose & cheeks. (5) *Miliaria* - obstructed sweat flow with rupture of eccrine sweat glands due to heat with 1-2 mm vesicle crops on uninflamed skin at intertriginous areas: scalp, face, trunk. (6) *Milia* - pearly yellow 1-3 mm papules on face of 50% newborns due to epidermal inclusion of pilosebaceous cyst of vellus hair.
Scaling dermatitides include (1) *irritant contact dermatitis* - red, scaling rash convex surfaces of perineum, lower abdomen, buttocks, & thighs sparing intertriginous areas. Secondary staphylococcal skin infection may occur. Treat with gentle cleaning, lubricants and barrier pastes (e.g., zinc oxide), and topical steroids. (2) *Candida* - bright red with sharp borders, satellite red papules and pustules, involves skin creases. Diagnose clinically or KOH slide and treat with topical antifungals. (3) *seborrheic dermatitis* - salmon colored patches with greasy yellow scales beginning in intertriginous areas, diaper, axilla and scalp (cradle cap). May persist up to 8-12 months old. Treat with mild keratolytics (e.g. antiseborrheic shampoos, zinc pyrithione, sulfur and salicylic acid topical preparation. Emollients, topical antifungals, and low potency topical steroids may resolve skin lesions.

Newborn Rashes continued...

Select serious diseases causing rashes in newborn period include (1) _congenital syphilis_ - skin lesions often begin between 2-6 weeks old with maculopapular eruption beginning on the palms and soles, later spreading to trunk. Smooth round, moist patches, involve the mouth and perianal area, while rhinitis with profuse and bloody rhinorrhea is often present. Systemic disease will manifest as lymphadenopathy, pneumonitis, nephritis, enteritis, pancreatitis, meningitis, or osteochondritis. (2) _Acrodermatitis enteropathica_ (AEP) - erosive diaper dermatitis, diarrhea, and hair loss during first few months of life. Weeping crusted red patches appear with a perioral, acral and intertrigenous distribution. Responds to oral/IV zinc. (3) _Herpes simplex_ - incubation period is 2-21 days (mean 6 days). Rash consists of 1-2 mm clustered papules and vesicles, becoming pustular & denuded. 1st lesions on scalp after head delivery. Multiorgan involvement common. Diagnose via Tzanck smear.

Childhood Exanthems

An exanthem is an eruption of skin associated with systemic illness.

Enteroviruses – > 30 exanthems are associated with coxsackie/ECHO viruses. Rash = maculopapular, scarlitiniform, vesicular or urticarial. (e.g. hand/foot/mouth – fever, malaise, then vesicles in mouth, on palms, feet, lasts 3-6 days, reoccurs.)

Erythema infectiosum _(5th disease)_ - Parvovirus B19 is the etiology. Seen in children aged 3-12. 30-60% attack rate. The rash begins with bright red cheeks, then later a faint maculopapular pink rash on the trunk and extremities, clearing in lacy pattern. Sunlight & warmth ↑ rash. Transient anemia & arthralgias may occur.

Roseola _(exanthem subitum)_ - Human herpes virus 6 is cause. Most common at 6 months to 3 years. Clinical course is characterized by sudden onset of high fever, periorbital puffiness, conjunctivitis, & occasionally a febrile seizure. Rash begins as fever declines. A faint pink, maculopapular (± pruritic) rash appears over trunk.

Rubella - Usually mild disease often causing subclinical illness. Main morbidity occurs through communicability (up to 7 days from onset of rash) to pregnant mother and fetus. URI prodrome with widespread lymphadenopathy, notably involving the postoccipital and postauricular nodes. Small macules coalesce on the trunk and fade by day three. Arthralgias are common.

Rubeola _(measles)_ - Begins with a prodrome of upper respiratory symptoms including cough, conjunctivitis, and coryza (nasal congestion). Exanthem begins 14 days after exposure, starting behind the ears and the hairline and spreading from head to feet. It is red and maculopapular with discrete lesions that become confluent. Pneumonia is most common reason for admission. Modified measles may develop in partially immune host (e.g., if received IgG) causing prolonged prodrome, and less ill appearance. Live vaccine given within 72 hr or ISG within 6 days of exposure prevents disease. Patients are infectious until 4h after rash onset.

Exanthems continued...

Scarlet fever - Reaction to toxin produced by Group A strep. pharyngitis 12-48 hours after onset sore throat. Rash is rough, blanches & appears 1st in skin folds (neck, groin, axilla, antecubitum). Circumoral pallor (sparing of area near mouth and nose). Without treatment, rash lasts 4-5 days with skin peeling on hands & feet over 2 weeks. 24 h of antibiotics are needed prior to being non-communicable.

Papulosquamous & Eczematous Rashes

Atopic Dermatitis – Dry scaling skin with intense pruritis. (1) <u>Acute</u> - erythema, scaling or tiny red vesicles that rupture/weep with scratching (2) <u>Subacute</u> – similar to acute with mild scaling, lichenification (3) <u>Chronic</u> – scaling, marked lichenification with minimal skin erythema. Excoriations are present in each stage. Location - < 2 years – acute/subacute lesions on cheeks, forehead, scalp, extensor surfaces of extremities. > 2 years – subacute/chronic lesions over flexural areas neck, elbows, wrists, knees, and ankles.

Atopic Dermatitis U.K. Working Party Diagnostic Criteria (itching + ≥ 3 ● features) *Br J Derm* 1994: 406.	● Itchy skin at elbows, knees, ankles, necks, OR if < 4 years cheek ● asthma or hayfever OR if < 4 years, atopy in a 1st degree relative	● Dry skin in past year ● Onset < 2 years old ● Visible flexural atopic dermatitis OR if < 4 years old, cheeks & forehead & outer limb

Chronic management – (1) Avoid irritants (2) Hydrate with tepid bath then emollient (e.g. *Aquaphor, Eucerin,* or *Cetaphil*) BID. (3) coal tar extract for lichenified non-inflammatory dermatitis. (e.g. *Liquor Carbonis Detergens* in *Aquaphor* or *Eucerin*) (4) <u>Acute flare up</u> *(a thru g)*– (a) ointment based <u>topical steroids</u>. Mild – 1% hydrocortisone, Moderate/Severe – fluticasone propionate (0.005% ointment *Cutivate*), mometasone furoate (0.1% cream/*Elocon*), prednicarbate (0.1% cream *Dermatop*) Avoid fluorinated & more potent steroids on face, intertriginous areas, and diaper area. (b) <u>antihistamine</u> - esp. at night. (c) <u>wet wraps</u> – apply topical steroid, then wrap area in cool wet towel for 10 min, remove towel, reapply steroid followed by application of moisturizer OR dress child in wet cotton pajama after applying topical steroid, then place dry pajama over wet one overnight. (d) <u>UV light</u> – (A&B) and psoralen or UVA, (e) <u>systemic steroid</u> taper – sparingly, only in adolescents, (f) <u>tacrolimus</u> (moderate-severe) or <u>pimecrolimus</u> (mild to moderate disease) ointment. (g) <u>cyclosporine</u> use short term & under close supervision.

Contact Dermatitis – due to irritants or allergens.

(1) *Diaper dermatitis* (irritant) - confluent erythema in areas of exposed moisture, friction (e.g. convex surfaces) & spares inguinal folds. Blistering & erosion may occur. Consider *Candida* infection if red intertriginous areas.

<u>Management</u> – (a) Keep area dry, (b) apply occlusive barrier (e.g. zinc oxide ointment after diaper change), (c) topical antifungal/steroid combination with occlusive barrier, (d) oral mycostatin, (e) treat breastfeeding mom's *Candida*.

Papulosquamous & Eczematous Rashes – continued...

(2) *Allergic dermatitis* exhibits initial eczematous reaction with red papules or
    vesicles overlying area of edema (e.g. linear streaks for poison ivy, oak,
    sumac). <u>Management</u> - remove offending agent, Burrow's solution, cool
    compresses, topical or brief systemic steroids.

Other Papulosquamous & Eczematous Rashes

Disorder & Treatment	Skin lesions	Location & Comments
Dyshidrotic eczema	Scaling vesicles, blisters fissures	Feet > hands, lateral digits, hyper-hidrosis ± localized atopic dermatitis
Eczema herpeticum *Acyclovir*	Herpes clusters at site of atopic dermatitis	If young patient, or more than mild involvement, IV *acyclovir*. If well appearing and older, PO acyclovir
Exfoliative dermatitis *Remove agent, treat underlying disease*	General erythema & scaling with exfoliation head to toe, fluid loss, bullae, & sepsis, + Nikolsky's sign	May be due to drugs (toxic epidermal necrolysis, e.g. penicillin, sulfa, phenobarbital, aspirin), dermatitides, immune disorder (e.g. HIV or Wiskott Aldrich), or leukemia/lymphoma
Pityriasis rosea	Papules, scales	Christmas tree pattern on trunk *(if African Am. may spare trunk)*
Psoriasis *Emollients, Topical steroids, UV light + Psoralen*	Round or oval red plaques with silvery scales	Scalp, trunk, extensor extremities, or areas of trauma. Nail pitting, dystrophy, and fissuring of palms and soles may be present.
Seborrheic dermatitis *Shampoo, Emollients, or Topical steroids*	Greasy scales, papules, erythema, pigment changes	Onset < 3 mo, disappears, reappears in adolesence. Hairbearing area face, scalp (cradle cap), axilla, inguinal areas, neck, post. to ear. Consider topical antifungals vs. *Pityrosporum*
Syphilis *IV Antibiotics Penicillin*	Maculopapular, de-squamation, vesicles, papules, warts, bullae	Maculopapular rash of palms/soles spreading to extremities & trunk; Moist warts (intertriginous, periorifice)
Tinea *Antifungals*	Red scales, papules, pustules, vesicles	Non-hair-bearing areas of scalp, trunk and extremities

Vesiculopustular Rashes

Rash	Skin lesions	Location
Impetigo	Honey colored crusting or bullae	Face, trunk, extremities
Staphylococcal scalded skin syndrome (SSSS)	Generalized sunburn, circumoral erythema, periorifice crusting, Nikolsky's sign, sterile bullae	Total body with sparing of mucous membranes. Primary site of infection may be conjunctivae, nasopharynx, intertriginous area, umbilical stump, or circumcision.
Herpes simplex	Grouped thick-walled vesicles, pustules	Face, trunk, extremities, perineum, or mucous membranes
Herpes zoster	Grouped papules, vesicles, erosions	Dermatomal distribution
Erythema multiforme	Papules, wheals, target lesions	Generalized, palms, soles, with ≥ 2 mucous membranes involved in Stevens - Johnson syndrome
Toxic epidermal necrolysis	Generalized sunburn, sloughing, Nikolsky's sign	Generalized with mucous membrane involvement. Deeper epidermal cleavage plane than SSSS

Other vesicular lesions – scabies, dyshidrosis, id reaction, insect bites, molluscum (simulates vesicles), Coxsackie (hand, foot, mouth)

Purpuric Rashes (also see Bleeding Disorders, pages 63-66)

Rash	Skin lesions	Location
Idiopathic thrombocytopenic purpura	Petechiae, ecchymoses, hematomas	Exposed sites, bony prominences, and mucosa
Acute leukemia	Petechiae, purpura	Generalized, with adenopathy, hepatosplenomegaly, sternal tenderness
Aplastic anemia	Petechiae, purpura, ecchymosis with thick raised centers	Generalized or sites of injury
DIC	Petechiae, purpura, areas of skin necrosis	Generalized (petechiae tend to be palpable with _meningococcemia_)
Factor deficiency (e.g., hemophilia)	Ecchymoses with thick raised centers	Exposed areas or sites of injury (petechiae unusual)

Other purpuric rashes: vasculitis, Rickettsia (RMSF), histiocytosis X, scurvy, trauma, medicines (steroids, thiazides), dysproteinemias, Kaposi's sarcoma, pyogenic granuloma.

Developmental Milestones

Age	Milestone
Newborn	• Lies flexed, turns head side to side, fixates to light and close objects
1 month	• More extended legs, responsive smile (6-8 weeks), follows object
4 months	• Lifts head/chest up, rolls front to back, reaches for objects, cooing
6 months	• Sits without support, pulls, bears some weight on legs, babbles
9 months	• Bears weight, stand holding on to furniture, crawls, says "mama/dada"
1 year	• Walks holding hand, pincer response, 3 words other than "mama"
2 years	• Climbs stairs, runs and jumps, uses spoon well, 3 word sentences
3 years	• Rides tricycle, briefly stands on foot, counts to 3, knows entire name
6 years	• Balances on foot, hops, counts to 10, 10 syllable sentences

Weight, Height, Head Circumference 5th, 50th, and 95th Percentiles

	Males				Females		
Age[1]	Height[2]	Weight[3]	HC[4]	Age[1]	Height[2]	Weight[3]	HC[4]
1 mo	50–55-59	3.2-4.3-5.4	35-37-40	1 mo	49-54-57	3.0-4.0-4.9	34-36-38
3 mo	57-61-65	4.4-6.0-7.4	38-41-43	3 mo	55-60-63	4.2-5.4-6.7	37-40-42
6 mo	63-68-72	6.2-7.9-9.5	42-44-46	6 mo	62-66-70	5.8-7.2-8.7	40-42-45
9 mo	68-72-77	7.5-9.2-10.9	44-46-48	9 mo	66-70-75	7-8.6-10.2	42-44-46
1 y	72-76-81	8.4-10.1-12	45-47-49	1 y	70-74-79	7.8-9.5-11	44-46-48
1.5 y	78-82-88	9.6-11.5-13.4	46-48-51	1.5 y	76-81-86	8.9-10.8-12.8	45-47-49
2 y	82-88-94	10.5-12.6-14.7	47-49-51	2 y	81-87-92	9.9-11.9-14.1	46-48-50
3 y	91-97-103	12.3-14.7-17.3	49-51-53	3 y	90-96-102	11.6-14-16.5	48-49-51
4 y	96-103-110	13.6-16.7-20.2	-	4 y	95-102-108	13.1-16-19.9	-
5 y	102-110-117	15.3-18.7-23.1	-	5 y	101-108-116	14.5-18-22.6	-

[1] y-years or mo-months, [2]Height-(cm), [3]Weight-kilograms, [4]HC- head circumference (cm)
United States Vital Statistics 1977 (Nov 165):I-IV; 1979: 1.

Other Growth Milestones

- *Dentition* – 1st teeth to erupt - lower incisors at 6 mo, central incisors (6-8 mo), lateral incisors (7-9 mo), 1st molar (12-14 mo), cuspids (16-18 mo), 2nd molars (20-24 mo). All 20 primary teeth erupt by 2 yr. Permanent teeth begin to erupt at 5-6 years, with all 32 erupting by teens.
- *Fontanelle* – Posterior fontanelle closes by 4 mo. Anterior fontanelle ↓in size at 6 mo, closes at 9-18 mo. (Testing required if ant. fontanelle open after 18 mo)
- *Sinuses* - The ethmoid and maxillary sinuses are aerated at birth, while the frontal and sphenoid sinuses become aerated at 5-6 years.
- *Menarche* – Mean age of menarche is 12.7 years (11-16 range).
  1. Precocious puberty - onset of menses before age 10
  2. Primary amenorrhea – absence of menses beyond 16 years (always abnormal and requires evaluation)

Adrenal Disorders

Adrenal Insufficiency

Fever, vomiting, altered mental status, ↓BP, shock, ↓Na+, ↑K+, ↓glucose. Associated with chronic steroid use or unidentified adrenal disease (e.g., Addison's, congenital enzyme defects).

Adrenal Crisis Therapy

- If possible, draw and store blood sample for later steroid-level analyses
- 20 ml/kg normal saline bolus IV to correct shock (may repeat as needed)
- Dextrose (see hypoglycemia, page 38) IV and hydrocortisone 1-2 mg/kg IV
- Antibiotics if suspicion of sepsis (e.g., ceftriaxone 50 mg/kg)
- DOCA (deoxycorticosterone acetate) 1-2 mg IM (less urgent than other treatments)

Diabetes Mellitus

Diabetic ketoacidosis (DKA)

DKA causes 70% of diabetic related deaths under the age of 10 years. DKA is the 1st presentation of diabetes in 15-30%.

Typical Deficits in DKA	Fluid	• 10% body weight (BW)
	Na+	• 8-10 mEq/kg of BW
	Cl-	• 5-7 mEq/kg of BW
	K+	• 5 mEq/kg of BW

Treatment of DKA

- Apply cardiac monitor and administer O_2 if altered mental status or shock.
- Replace fluid and electrolyte deficits gradually over the first 24-48 hours.
- **The 1st hour**: Normal saline 10-20 ml/kg IV bolus (repeat prn to correct shock) Load insulin 0.1 units/kg IV (some experts avoid bolus and begin with drip).
- **1-9 hours**: After correcting hypotension, administer 50% of fluid deficit with 0.45% NS over next 8 hours. Consider 0.9% NS if 1st serum Na+ < 135 mEq/L.
- **10-24 hours**: Replace the remaining 50% fluid deficit over this time period.
- **Add dextrose** to the IV fluids when the glucose falls to < 250-300 mg/dl.
- **Replace K+** (if OK urine output) and phosphate. Phosphate shifts O_2 dissociation curve to the right (increasing O_2 delivery to tissues and correcting acidosis). Replace K+ with approximately 50/50 mix of KCL and K_3PO_4.

If serum potassium is	Potassium in IV fluids
<3 mEq/l	40-60 mEq/l
3-4 mEq/l	30 mEq/l
4-5 mEq/l	20 mEq/l
5-6 mEq/l	< 10 mEq/l

- **Insulin:** Infusion of approximately 0.1 units/kg/hour. Change to subcutaneous insulin when pH >7.30 and monitor hourly glucose. If glucose drops to 250 mg/dl, reduce the rate of insulin administration to 0.02-0.05 units/kg/hour.

Criteria for outpatient treatment of DKA

- Initial glucose <500 and *either* a pH ≥ 7.2 or a bicarbonate ≥ 10 mEq/L (have > 90% chance of resolving metabolic parameters within 3 hours.)
- pH ≥ 7.35 and bicarbonate ≥ 20 mEq/L after 3 hours of treatment
- Resolution of significant symptoms and vital sign abnormalities
- Reliable parents, older patient, and closely coordinated follow-up

Am J Dis Child 1988; 142:448

Other Complications of Diabetes and Therapy

- *Cerebral edema* is unpredictable in onset with ↓ mental status, coma, and pupillary changes 8-12 h after initiation of therapy. Associated with bicarbonate administration, initial low pCO$_2$, high BUN, & not amount of fluid administered. Mortality is > 90%. Treat with mannitol, intubation, and hyperventilation.
- *Hyperosmolar coma* is very rare in children and is associated with preexisting neurologic disorders. Fluids and management of underlying cause are primary treatment modalities. Only 10-50% of the insulin dose used in DKA is needed.

Hypoglycemia

Hypoglycemia is defined as a blood glucose < 40-45 mg/dl (< 30 mg/dl in neonate). Hypoglycemia is ketotic in > 50% case. It is most commonly due to poor nutrition or overmedication with insulin or hypoglycemic agents.

Etiology of Hypoglycemia

• ↓ Intake (vomiting, malnutrition)	• Excess endogenous insulin (e.g., islet cell tumors)
• ↓Absorption (diarrhea, malabsorption)	
• Inborn errors of metabolism (amino acid, glycogen storage, or glucose metabolic enzyme deficiencies)	• Insulin or oral hypoglycemic excess
	• Endocrine disorder: Hypopituitarism, hypothyroidism, adrenal insufficiency
• Sepsis, Reye's syndrome	• Poison (aspirin, β-blockers, alcohol)

Evaluation

History: Fed hypoglycemia (< 4-6 h after meal) is associated with GI tract disease (poor absorption), and early diabetes while *fasting hypoglycemia* (> 5-6 h after meal) is associated with insulin secreting tumors, and endocrine disorders.
Dipstick urine for ketones. Absence of ketones suggests hyperinsulinemia (medication or tumor) or defect in fatty acid oxidation.

Management of Hypoglycemia

Age	Dose and Concentration	Other Treatment[1]
0-30 days	• 10 ml/kg of D$_{10}$W IV	• glucagon 0.02-0.03 mg/kg if < 20kg; 1 mg if > 20 kg administer IM, SC, or IV
1-24 months	• 4 ml/kg of D$_{25}$W IV	
> 2 years	• 2 ml/kg of D$_{50}$W IV	• diazoxide IV if severe

[1]Octreotide may be used IV if hyperinsulinemia or sulfonylurea overdose.

Environmental Disorders

Minor Heat Illness

- *Heat Syncope*: Postural hypotension from vasodilation, volume depletion, & ↓ vascular tone. Rehydrate, remove from heat, and evaluate for serious disease.
- *Heat Cramps*: Painful, contractions of calves, thigh, or shoulders in those who are sweating liberally and drinking hypotonic solutions (e.g. water). Replace fluids: 0.1-0.2% NS oral solution or IV NS rehydration. Do not use salt tablets.
- *Heat Exhaustion*: Salt and water depletion causing orthostasis, and hyperthermia (usually < 104F). Mental status and neurologic exam are normal. Lab: high hematocrit, high sodium, or high BUN. Treat with NS 10-20 ml/kg IV.

Heatstroke

Clinical Features	Risk Factors
• Hyperpyrexia (temp. > 104-105.8F) • Central nervous system dysfunction (seizures, altered mentation, plantar responses, hemiplegia, ataxia) • Loss of sweating (variably present)	• Very young or old age • Drugs that limit sweating (anticholinergics, amphetamines, cocaine, antihypertensive agents)

Complications of heatstroke: rhabdomyolysis, renal or liver failure, ↓ Na, ↓ Ca, ↓ phosphate, ↓ or ↑K and disseminated intravascular coagulation.

Management of Heatstroke

- Administer oxygen, protect airway if comatose or seizing. Check blood glucose.
- Measure temperature with continuous rectal probe accurate at high levels.
- Begin IV NS cautiously as pulmonary edema is common and mean fluid requirement is < 20 ml/kg in 1st 4 hours. Consider central line pressures as guide.
- Immediate cooling by: (1) *evaporation*: Spray with tepid water and direct fan at patient (0.1 - 0.3C/min temp. drop).   For shivering, IV lorazepam 0.05-0.1 mg/kg IV or (2) *ice water (or 60F) tub immersion: (controversial)* (temp. drop ~ 0.16C/min). (3) *Ice packs, cooling blankets, peritoneal dialysis, gastric lavage* with cold water are slow or unproven. (4) Avoid aspirin (hyperpyrexia). Avoid repeat acetaminophen doses (possible liver damage & ineffective in heatstroke).
- Stop above measures at temperature of 102-104 to avoid over-correction.
- Place Foley catheter to monitor urine output (see rhabdomyolysis page 40).
- Obtain CBC, electrolytes, renal function, glucose, liver enzymes, LDH/CPK, PT, and PTT, arterial blood gas, and fibrin degradation products. ECG and CXR.
- Exclude other fever cause: infection, malignant hyperthermia, thyroid, drugs, etc

Other Heat Related Disorders

- **Malignant Hyperthermia (MH)** : Autosomal dominant. Fever, + muscle rigidity after anesthetics or succinylcholine. *Treatment*: Stop agent, lower temperature as in heatstroke (avoid phenothiazines), give dantrolene 2-3 mg/kg IV (max 10 mg/kg).

- **Neuroleptic Malignant Syndrome:** Similar to MH with fever, muscle rigidity, and altered mentation, but due to anticholinergics (e.g. phenothiazines). *Treatment:* Stop agent, treat heatstroke (avoid phenothiazines) and administer dantrolene 2-3 mg/kg IV (max 10 mg/kg) and bromocriptine 2.5-10 mg PO tid.

- **Rhabdomyolysis:** Syndrome with release of contents into circulation due to tissue hypoxia, direct injury, exercise, enzyme defects, metabolic disease (DKA, $\downarrow$K, $\downarrow$ Na, or $\downarrow$ phosphate, thyroid), toxins, infections, heatstroke. *Complications:* renal failure, $\uparrow$K, $\uparrow$Ca or $\downarrow$ Ca, $\uparrow$or$\downarrow$phosphate, $\uparrow$ uric acid, compartment syndrome, DIC. *Treatment:* (1) IV NS to keep UO^1 > 2-3 ml/kg/hr, (2) Alkalinize urine, (3) Mannitol if poor UO: 0.25-0.5 g/kg IV, + add 12.5 g to each L NS, (4) Dialyze $\uparrow$K$^+$, or uremia.

UO^1 – urine output

HYPOTHERMIA

Severity	Temp. F (C)	Features
Mild	91-95 (33-35)	Maximal shivering + slurred speech at < 95°F
Moderate	85-90 (29-32)	At < 89°F altered mental status, mydriasis, shivering ceases, muscles are rigid, incoordination, bradypnea
Severe	$\leq$ 82 ($\leq$ 28)	Bradycardia in 50%, Osborne waves on ECG, voluntary motion stops, pupils are fixed and dilated
	79 (26)	Loss of consciousness, areflexia, no pain response
	77 (25)	No respirations, appear dead, pulmonary edema
	68 (20)	Asystole

Management of Hypothermia

- No vigorous manipulation or active external rewarming unless mild hypothermia
- Evaluate for cause (e.g. sepsis, hypoglycemia, CNS disease, adrenal crisis).
- **Mild hypothermia** (> 32°C): Administer humidified warmed O$_2$. Passive external rewarming and treatment of underlying disease is often only treatment needed.
- **Moderate hypothermia** (29-32°C): Active internal rewarming. Drugs & cardioversion for cardiac arrest may be ineffective. Warm humidified O$_2$, with gastric or peritoneal lavage if < 1C/hour temperature rise. Perform CPR, and advanced life support prn.
- **Severe hypothermia** ($\leq$ 29°C): (1) Warm humidified O$_2$, and warm IV fluids. (2) If nonarrested, warmed peritoneal dialysis (41C dialysate), or (3) pleural irrigation (41C). (4) If core temperature < 25C consider femoral-femoral bypass. (5) Use open pleural lavage for direct cardiac rewarming if core temp < 28C after 1 h of bypass in an arrest rhythm. If signs of life, & non-arrested, avoid CPR & ACLS. (6) If cardiac arrest, CPR and ACLS are OK. (7) Do not treat atrial arrhythmias. (8) Use NS to treat $\downarrow$BP. Use pressors cautiously prn. (8) Consider D$_{10}$/D$_{25}$, naloxone, hydrocortisone 1 mg/kg IV.

Snake Bite Envenomation

Grade	Features of Crotalidae Envenomation	Equine Antivenin dose
None	± Fang marks, no pain, erythema or systemic symptoms	None
Mild	Fang marks, mild pain/edema, no systemic symptoms	0-5 vials (50 ml)
Moderate	Fang marks, severe pain, moderate edema in 1st 12 h, mild symptoms (vomiting, paresthesias), mild coagulopathy (without bleeding)	10 vials (100 ml)
Severe	Fang marks, severe pain/edema, severe symptoms (↓BP, respiratory distress), coagulopathy with bleeding	15-20 vials (150-200 ml)

Emergency Treatment for Crotalid Envenomation

- Decrease movement, and immobilize extremity at or below level of heart.
- Avoid incision & drainage and tourniquets.
- Perform exam, measure envenomation site, and administer fluids, pressors prn.
- If no signs of envenomation, clean wound, administer tetanus and observe for a minimum of 6 hours. Consider antibiotics (e.g. *Augmentin* X 5 days).
- If significant envenomation, obtain CBC, electrolytes, renal and liver function tests, PT, PTT, fibrinogen, urinalysis, ECG, and type and cross.
- Choose Equine or Ovine Antivenom based on availability. Ovine is preferred although it has not been well studied ≤ 8 years old.

Ovine - Crotalidae Polyvalent Immune Fab Antivenin (FabAV)

- Sheep derived more potent than equine antivenom with less allergy.
- Regardless of grade administer initial dose of 6 vials.
- Administer an additional 2 vials at 6, 12, and 18 hours.
- Dilute FabAV to a total of 250 ml in NS (if > 10 kg) & infuse IV over one hour.
- Protherics Inc., the manufacturer of CroFab, states "the absolute venom dose is expected to be the same in children & adults, therefore, no dosage adjustment for age should be made". www.protherics.com *Ann Emerg Med* 2001; 37:181.

Equine - Antivenin Crotalidae Polyvalent Administration - see dose above

- Skin test only if equine to be administered: 0.2 ml SC (dilute 1:10 with NS) distant from bite. Observe ≥ 10 min. Absent reaction does not exclude allergy.
- Need for antivenin and specific dose is controversial. Prior to administration, obtain consent, administer 1% NS, consider premedication with diphenhydramine 1 mg/kg IV, and dilute antivenom in 50-100 ml each vial.
- Reconstitute antivenin in a 1:10 solution with NS or D_5W.
- Administer 5-10 ml over 5 min. If no allergy, increase rate so that infusion takes 1-2 hours. If symptoms progress, additional antivenin may be required.
- If allergic reaction & antivenin is necessary, consider arterial line continue to treat with NS ± albumin, methylprednisolone 1-2 mg/kg IV, and diphenhydramine 0.5-1.0 mg/kg IV. Hang epinephrine drip in line separate from antivenin (see page 191), & maximally dilute antivenin. Begin antivenin slowly. If needed begin epi drip at low dose [1 ml/hr of above ~ 0.1 μg/kg/min] Once allergic reaction gone, restart antivenin slowly. Contact poison center.

Elapidae (Coral Snake) Envenomation

Southeast US and Arizona. These snakes must bite & chew. Local effects + bite marks may be minimal. Symptoms are systemic: altered LOC, cranial nerve deficits, weakness/respiratory failure and may be delayed 24 h. Admit for respiratory or neurologic deterioration. All require Coral Snake Antivenin. *Dose of antivenin*: 3-6 vials administered as crotalidae antivenin. Sonoran (Arizona) coral snake venom is less toxic, no deaths have been reported, and coral snake antivenin is ineffective.

Special Situations

Mojave rattlesnake: May cause muscle weakness, paralysis, or respiratory failure with few local symptoms. Crotalidae Polyvalent Immune Fab (Ovine) is effective, Antivenin Crotalidae Polyvalent is not.

Exotic snakes: Call **(602) 626-6016** for information regarding available antivenin.

Serum sickness will develop in many receiving > 5 vials of antivenin within 5-20 days causing joint pain, myalgias, and possibly rash. Warn patient and treat with diphenhydramine (*Benadryl*) 1 mg/kg PO q4-6 h and prednisone 1-2 mg/kg PO qd.

Spider Bites

Black Widow Spiders	Features of Black Widow Bites
• Found in all of US, mostly South	• Mild to moderately painful bite,
• Females ~ 5 cm with legs and 1.5 cm without legs	• In 1hour, redness, swelling, & cramping at bite which later spread.
• Only females are toxic	• Abd. wall pain mimics peritonitis
• 1/5 have red hour glass on abdomen	• $\downarrow$BP, shock, coma, resp. failure

Management of Black Widow Spider Bites	
• Lorazepam *Ativan* 0.05-0.1 mg/kg IV	Indications[1] for Admission/Antivenin
• Consider Antivenin – Dose: 1-2 vials IV in 50-100 ml NS Skin test prior to using	• Respiratory or cardiac symptoms • Severe cramping or pain despite calcium and lorazepam use
• Allergy & serum sickness can occur	• History of $\uparrow$ BP or cardiac disease
• Calcium is ineffective	

[1]controversial as no deaths have occurred in 30 years *Emerg Med Clin North Am* 1992; 269

Brown Recluse Spiders	Management
• Live mostly in southern US. Bites are mild or painless.	• Wound care, tetanus
• At 1st, lesions are red and blanch	• Consider excising if > 2 cm & well-circumscribed border (usually 2 to 3 weeks after bite)
• Later a macule, ulcer or blister	• ± Hyperbaric oxygen (controversial)
• Arthralgias, GI upset, DIC, or shock	
• Hemoglobinuria (renal failure)	

Marine Envenomation

↙ Puncture Wounds ↘

Sea snakes, blue ring octupus cone shells	Starfish, sea urchin, stingrays, catfish weeverfish, scorpionfish
↓	↓
Lymphatic venous occlusion and pressure immobilization	• Immerse in hot water (45C) X 30-90 min or until pain subsides • Irrigate, after local/regional anesthesia • Debride + obtain xray to look for spine
↓	
Supportive and respiratory care Sea snake antivenin[1,3]	Provide supportive care and administer Stone fish (scorpionfish) antivenin[2,3]

[1] **_Sea snakes_**. Bites are painless, causing paralysis + muscle necrosis. Administer polyvalent sea snake antivenin (Commonwealth Serum Lab, Australia) within 36 h. If unavailable, Tiger snake and polyvalent _Elapidae_ antivenin are effective.

[2] **_Stone fish (a type of scorpionfish)_**. Venom causes muscle toxicity, with paralysis of cardiac, skeletal, and involuntary muscles. Pain is immediate and intense. The wound is ischemic, cyanotic and may lose tissue. Heat (45C) partially inactivates venom. Follow package insert for antivenin (Commonwealth Serum Labs, Australia).

[3] In US, call **(619) 222-6363** or **(415) 770-7171** for antivenin.

↙ Marine Exposures Causing Urticaria or Vesicles ↘

Hydroids, fire coral, jellyfish, anemones	Sponges, bristleworms
• Apply acetic acid 5%, isopropyl alcohol, 40-70%, or baking soda x 30 min • Remove nematocysts with forceps[1]	Extract spicules, with adhesive tape
↓	↓
	Acetic acid 5% or isopropyl alcohol
• Supportive care for systemic reaction • Antivenin for box jellyfish, C. flexneri • Consider systemic steroids	• Topical steroids if mild reaction • Treat for allergic reactions

[1] Do not rinse in fresh water.

Marine Infections

- Organisms causing soft tissue infection: _Aeromonas hydrophilia, B. fragilis, E. coli, Pseudomonas, Salmonella, Vibrio, Staph./Strep. species, C. perfringens._
- Irrigate, debride, explore, and obtain x-rays to exclude foreign bodies
- Antibiotic agents for treating soft tissue infection or prophylaxis:
  <u>Parenteral agents</u> - 3rd generation cephalosporin and/or an aminoglycoside
  <u>Oral agents</u> -_Septra_, cefuroxime, tetracycline if > 8-12 years.

Electrolyte Disorders

Formulas

Anion Gap	• $Na^+ - (Cl^- + HCO_3^-)$ *Normal = 8-16 mEq/L*
Osmolal gap	• measured – calculated osmolality *Normal = 0-10 mOsm/L*
Calculated Osmolality	• $2 \times Na^+ + (glucose/18) + (BUN/2.8) + (ethanol/4.6) + (methanol/2.6) + (ethylene glycol/5) + (acetone/5.5) + (isopropanol/5.9)$

See Page 95 for Evaluation Organic Acidurias and other Metabolic Disorders

Causes of ↑Anion Gap		Causes of ↓Anion Gap	Cause of ↑Osmol Gap
Methanol Uremia Diabetes Paraldehyde Iron, INH	Lactate Ethanol, ethylene glycol Salicylates, starvation	Lithium, Multiple myeloma Albumin loss in nephrotic syndrome	Alcohols (methanol, ethylene glycol, isopropanol) Sugars (glycerol, mannitol) Ketones (acetone)

	Primary Disorder	Normal Compensation
Acid Base Rules of Compensation	Metabolic Acidosis	$PCO_2 = (1.5 \times HCO_3^- + 8) \pm 2$
	Acute Respiratory Acidosis	$\uparrow \Delta HCO_3^- = (0.1 \times \Delta PCO_2 \uparrow)$
	Chronic Respiratory Acidosis	$\uparrow \Delta HCO_3^- = (0.4 \times \Delta PCO_2 \uparrow)$
	Metabolic Alkalosis	$PCO_2 = (0.9 \times HCO_3^- + 9) \pm 2$
	Acute Respiratory Alkalosis	$\downarrow \Delta HCO_3^- = (0.2 \times \Delta PCO_2 \downarrow)$
	Chronic Respiratory Alkalosis	$\downarrow \Delta HCO_3^- = (0.4 \times \Delta PCO_2 \downarrow)$

High Yield Criteria for Electrolyte Ordering in the ED	• Age ≤ 6 months • Vomiting • Tachycardia	• Diabetes mellitus • Dry mucous membranes • Capillary refill > 2 seconds

Presence of any criteria was 100% sensitive in detecting significant abnormalities.
Acad Emerg Med 1997; 4:1025.

CALCIUM

Hypocalcemia - Total calcium < 8.5 mg/dl or ionized Ca^{+2} < 2.0 mEq/L (1.0 mmol/L)
Hypercalcemia - Total calcium > 10.5 mg/dl or ionized Ca^{+2} > 2.7 mEq/L (1.3 mmol/L)

Hypoalbuminemia correction	• For each change in serum albumin of 1 g/dl ↑ or ↓, serum calcium changes 0.8 mg/dl in same direction

Hypocalcemia – Clinical Features

Symptoms	Physical Findings	Electrocardiogram
Paresthesias, fatigue Seizures, tetany Vomiting, weakness Laryngospasm	Hyperactive reflexes Chvostek(C)/Trousseau(T) signs[1] Low blood pressure Congestive heart failure	• Prolonged QT (esp. Ca^{+2} < 6.0 mg/dl) • Bradycardia • Arrhythmias

[1]C–muscle twitch with tap facial nerve, T–carpal spasm after forearm BP cuff up for 3 min

Hypocalcemia Etiology [1,2]

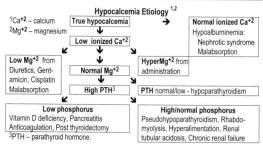

[1]Ca^{+2} – calcium
[2]Mg^{+2} – magnesium

True hypocalcemia →

Normal ionized Ca^{+2}
Hypoalbuminemia:
Nephrotic syndrome
Malabsorption

Low ionized Ca^{+2}

Low Mg^{+2} from
Diuretics, Gent-
amicin, Cisplatin
Malabsorption

Normal Mg^{+2}

HyperMg^{+2} from
administration

High PTH[3]

PTH normal/low - hypoparathyroidism

Low phosphorus
Vitamin D deficiency, Pancreatitis
Anticoagulation, Post thyroidectomy
[3]PTH – parathyroid hormone.

High/normal phosphorus
Pseudohypoparathyroidism, Rhabdomyolysis, Hyperalimentation, Renal
tubular acidosis, Chronic renal failure

Drugs That Cause Hypocalcemia

- Cimetidine
- Cisplatin
- Citrate (transfusion)
- Dilantin, phenobarbital
- Gentamicin, Tobramycin
- Glucagon
- Glucocorticoids
- Heparin
- Loop diuretics (*Lasix*)
- Magnesium sulfate
- Phosphates
- Protamine
- Norepinephrine
- Na nitroprusside
- Theophylline

Hypocalcemia Treatment

Check serum electrolytes, BUN, creatinine, albumin, magnesium, arterial pH			
Drug	Preparation	Route	Drug Dose (max. dose)[3]
Ca gluconate	10% solution –100mg/ml	IM, IV[1,2]	0.5-1 ml/kg (5-10 ml)
Ca chloride	10% solution –100mg/ml	IV[1,2]	0.2-0.3 ml/kg (5-10 ml)
Ca gluconate	500, 650, 975, 1000mg	PO	100 mg/kg qid (500 mg/kg)

[1] Administer IV calcium (Ca) slowly (over ≥ 5-10 min) while patient on cardiac monitor. IV calcium may cause hypotension, tissue necrosis, bradycardia or digoxin toxicity.

[2] Consider central administration to prevent tissue damage. Local infiltration of hyaluronidase reverses necrosis.

[3] All are doses of salt (listed drug) and not of pure elemental calcium.

Hypercalcemia – Clinical Features

General	•	Weakness, polydipsia, dehydration
Neurologic	•	Confusion, irritability, hyperreflexia, headache
Skeletal	•	Bone pain, fractures
Cardiac	•	Hypertension, QT shortening, wide T wave, arrhythmia
GI	•	Anorexia, weight loss, constipation, ulcer, pancreatitis
Urologic	•	Polyuria, renal insufficiency, nephrolithiasis

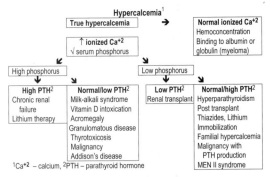

Hypercalcemia[1]

True hypercalcemia	→	Normal ionized Ca^{+2}

High PTH[2] — Chronic renal failure, Lithium therapy

Normal/low PTH[2] — Milk-alkali syndrome, Vitamin D intoxication, Acromegaly, Granulomatous disease, Thyrotoxicosis, Malignancy, Addison's disease

Low PTH[2] — Renal transplant

Normal/high PTH[2] — Hyperparathyroidism, Post transplant, Thiazides, Lithium, Immobilization, Familial hypercalcemia, Malignancy with PTH production, MEN II syndrome

[1]Ca^{+2} – calcium, [2]PTH – parathyroid hormone

Hypercalcemia Management

• Especially important for Ca^{+2} > 12 mg/dl, hypotension, or cardiac arrhythmias
• IV NS 20 ml/kg with repeat boluses to keep urine output > 2-3 ml/kg/hour
• Furosemide 1-2 mg/kg to promote urinary calcium excretion (after adequate hydration)
• Consider IV hydrocortisone (1-2 mg/kg) if sarcoid, vitamin A or D toxicity, or leukemia, mithramycin (metastatic bone disease). Calcitonin and dialysis may also be useful

MAGNESIUM

<u>Hypomagnesemia</u> (<1.5 mEq/L) Due to diuretics, aminoglycosides, cyclosporine. Irritable muscle, tetany, seizure, arrhythmia. <u>Treat</u>: $MgSO_4$ 25-50 mg/kg IV over 20 min.
<u>Hypermagnesemia</u> (>2.2 mEq/L) Due to renal failure, excess maternal Mg supplement, or overuse of Mg-containing medicine. Clinical features: weakness, hyporeflexia, paralysis, and ECG with AV block & QT prolongation. <u>Treat</u>: $CaCl$ (10%) 0.2-0.3 ml/kg (max 5 ml) IV.

POTASSIUM

Acute decreases in pH will increase K^+ (a ↓pH of 0.1 will ↑K^+ 0.3-1.3 mEq/L). Acute metabolic acid base disorders cause most changes.

Hypokalemia
Causes of Hypokalemia

• *Decreased K^++ intake* • *Intracellular shift* (normal stores): alkalemia, insulin, pseudohypo-kalemia of leukemia, familial hypo-kalemic periodic paralysis (HPP).	• *Increased excretion*: diuretics, hyper-aldosteronism, penicillins (exchange Na^+/K^+), sweating, diarrhea (colonic fluid has high K^+), vomiting (compensation for metabolic alkalosis)

Clinical Features of Hypokalemia	Treatment of Hypokalemia
• Lethargy, confusion, weakness • Areflexia, difficult respirations • Autonomic instability, Low BP	• Ensure good urine output first • If mild, replace orally only • Parenteral K^+ if severe hypokalemia
ECG findings in Hypokalemia	(e.g. cardiac or neuromuscular
• $K^+ \le 3.0$ mEq/L: low voltage QRS, flat T waves, ↓ ST segment, prominent P and U waves. • $K^+ \le 2.5$ mEq/L: prominent U wave • $K^+ \le 2.0$ mEq/L: widened QRS	symptoms or DKA). • Administer K^+ no faster than 0.5-1.0 mEq/kg/hour using ≤ 40 mEq/L (cautiously while continuously on cardiac monitor)

Hyperkalemia

Causes of Hyperkalemia	
• *Pseudohyperkalemia* due to blood samples or hemolysis • *Exogenous:* blood, salt substitutes, K^+ containing drugs (e.g. penicillin derivatives), acute digoxin toxicity, β blockers, succinylcholine	• *Endogenous* – acidemia, trauma, burns, rhabdomyolysis, DIC, sickle cell crisis, GI bleed, chemotherapy (destroying tumor mass), mineralo-corticoid deficiency, congenital defects (21 hydroxylase deficiency)

Clinical Features of Hyperkalemia	Treatment of Hyperkalemia
• Paresthesias, weakness • Ascending paralysis sparing head, trunk, and respiration • Life threatening arrhythmias	• Calcium chloride (10%) to stabilize membrane – 0.1-0.3 ml/kg (max 5 ml) IV over 2-5 min. Same dose may be repeated q 5 min x 2 more doses.
ECG in Hyperkalemia (K^+ in mEq/L)	• $NaHCO_3$ 1-2 mEq/kg IV, may repeat
• K^+ 5-6.0: peak T waves • K^+ 6-6.5: ↑ PR and QT intervals • K^+ 6.5-7: ↓P, ↓ ST segments • K^+ 7-7.5: ↑intraventricular conduction • K^+ 7.5-8: ↑QRS widens, ST and T waves merge • K^+ > 10: sine wave appearance	• Glucose 0.5-1.0 g/kg IV + insulin 1 unit/3g glucose IV (transcellular shift) • Albuterol nebulizer 1 cc, may repeat • Furosemide 1 mg/kg IV • Kayexalate 1 g/kg orally or rectally (lowers K^+ 1.2 mEq/L in 4-6 hours) • Dialysis

SODIUM

Daily Na^+ requirements: 1-2 mEq/kg/d in newborn and 3-4 mEq/kg/d - premature.
FE_{Na} = fraction of Na^+ in urine filtered by the glomerulus and not reabsorbed.
FE_{Na} = 100 x (urine Na^+/plasma Na^+) / (urine creatinine/plasma creatinine)
Normal FE_{Na} is < 3%, except under 2 months of age when FE_{Na} up may be to 5%.

Hyponatremia

Pseudohyponatremia occurs with ↑glucose, ↑triglyceride and ↑protein.

Na^+ = falsely ↓ 1.6 mEq/L for each 100 mg/dL ↑ in glucose over 100 mg/dL.

Clinical Features of Hyponatremia	
• Lethargy, apathy	• Cerebral edema
• Depressed reflexes, muscle cramps	• Seizures
• Pseudobulbar palsies	• Hypothermia

Hyponatremia Etiology, Diagnosis, Management

Deficit body Na^+ > deficit body water		Excess total body water (no edema)	Excess total body water > excess Na^+ (edema)	
↓	↓	↓	↓	↓
Renal losses: diuretics, mineralocorticoid deficiency, salt losing nephritis, bicarbonaturia, ketonuria, osmotic diuresis	*Extrarenal loss:* vomit, diarrhea, 3rd space fluids, pancreatitis, peritonitis, traumatized muscle	Glucocorticoid deficiency, low thyroid, pain, emotional stress, drugs, (SIADH - U_{osm} usually > S_{osm})	Nephrotic syndrome, cirrhosis, CHF	Acute and chronic renal failure
↓	↓	↓	↓	↓

Diagnostic Tests				
Na^+>20 mEq/L ↑FE_{Na}, ↓ SG^1 U_{osm}^3 varies	Na^+<10 mEq/L ↓FE_{Na}, ↑ SG^1 U_{osm}^3 > 800	Na^+>20 mEq/L Nl^2 FE_{Na}, ↑ SG^1 U_{osm}^3 varies	Na^+<10 mEq/L ↓FE_{Na}, ↑ SG^1 high U_{osm}^3	Na^+>20 mEq/L ↑FE_{Na}, ↓ SG^1 U_{osm}^3 varies
↓	↓	↓	↓	↓

Management				
Isotonic saline	Isotonic saline	Water restrict	Water restrict	Water restrict

[1] SG – specific gravity, [2] Nl – normal, [3] U_{osm} – urine osmolality, [4] S_{osm} – serum osmolality

Hypertonic Saline Administration
• Only use if severe ↓ Na^+(<120 mEq/L) with seizures, or other life threats
• Administer 4 ml/kg 3% saline, at ≤ 1-2 ml/kg/hour OR bolus over 20 minutes
• 1 ml/kg of 3% saline raises serum Na by 1 mEq/L

Hypernatremia

Clinical Features of Hypernatremia	
• Lethargy, irritability, coma	• Doughy skin
• Seizures	• Late preservation of intravascular
• Spasticity, hyperreflexia	volume (and vital signs)

Hypernatremia Etiology, Diagnosis, Management[1]

Na⁺ + H₂0 loss with low total body Na⁺		H₂0 loss with normal total body Na⁺		Excess Na⁺ with increased total body Na⁺
Renal losses osmotic diuresis (mannitol, glucose, urea)	*Extrarenal loss* excess sweat, diarrhea	*Renal loss* diabetes insipidus (nephrogenic, central) Serum osm > 295 mosm/L, Serum Na+ > 145 mEq/L, U_{osm} < 150 mosm./L	*Extrarenal loss* Respiratory and skin loss	Primary hyperaldosteronism, Cushing's syndrome, hypertonic dialysis, hypertonic bicarbonate, NaCl tablets

Diagnostic Tests

U Na⁺>20 mEq/L, U_{osm} hypotonic	U Na⁺<10 mEq/L, U_{osm} > 600-800 mosm/L	U Na⁺ varies U_{osm} often < 100-150 mosm/L	U Na⁺ varies U_{osm} > 600-800 mOsm/L	U Na⁺>20 mEq/L U_{osm} isotonic or hypertonic

Management

Hypotonic saline	Hypotonic saline	Water replacement D_5W	Water replacement D_5W	Diuretic+H₂0 replacement D_5W

[1] U-urine, U_{osm} – urine osmolality

Management of Hypernatremia

- Correct hypernatremia slowly over approximately 48 hours. Overvigorous rehydration causes cerebral edema, seizures, coma, or death. Lower Na⁺ no faster than 1-2 mEq/L/hour.
- With endogenous Na⁺ overload, treatment consists of salt restriction and correction of the primary underlying disorder. If there is excess exogenous mineralocorticoid, restrict salt and modify replacement therapy.
- Desmopressin (DDAVP) is indicated in children with diabetes insipidus. Intranasal DDAVP dose - 1.25-10 µg q day or bid.

Fluid Homeostasis

Clinical Findings in Dehydration

Findings	Mild(<5%)	Moderate (5-9%)	Severe (≥10%)
appearance	alert	restless	limp,cold, acrocyanosis
heart rate	normal	rapid weak	thready
respirations	normal	deep, increased	deep and rapid
blood pressure	normal	normal or low	low
skin turgor	normal	slow retraction	retraction > 2 sec
eyes	normal	sunken	grossly sunken
tears	present	absent	absent
mucous membranes	moist	dry	very dry
urine output	normal	reduced, dark	minimal
urine specific gravity	≤ 1.020	~ 1.030	> 1.035
BUN	normal	elevated	very high
arterial pH	> 7.30	7.00 - 7.30	< 7.10
fluid deficit	40-50 ml/kg	60-90 ml/kg	100 ml/kg or more

Dehydration – Classification and Management

Classification	Isotonic	Hypotonic	Hypertonic[1]
Na^+ (mEq/L)	130-150	< 130	> 150
Cause	Usually GI[2] and ECF[2] fluid loss	Dilute fluid (water) replacement	Too dilute formula, ↑ Na^+ in, ICF>ECF[3] loss.
Deficit	Na^+ = water loss	Na^+ > water loss	Water > Na^+ loss
Examination			
BP	Depressed	Very depressed	May be preserved
HR	Increased	Increased	Minimal increase
Turgor	Poor	Very poor	Fair
Skin	Dry	Clammy	Doughy
Mentation	Lethargy	Coma or seizure	Irritable or seizure
Rehydrate[4]	Normal saline	Normal saline	D_5 ½NS with K^+
Unique Feature	Most common. Oral rehydration is appropriate for children if< 5-10% dehydration if able to take liquids PO	Consider 3% NS if severe, life-threatening symptoms (see page 48 for indications and dosing)	NS can paradoxically ↑ Na^+. Lower Na^+ < 2 mEq/L/h or < 10 mEq /L/d. Too rapid Rx = CHF, CNS edema, renal damage.±↓Ca^{+2}
Exclude hypoglycemia in all patients.			

[1] Four ml/kg free water deficit for each 1 mEq/L Na > 145. [2]GI – gastrointestinal, [3]ICF – intracellular fluid, ECF – extracellular fluid, [4] Use NS to reverse shock in all cases

Detection of dehydration	High Yield Criteria > 5% dehydration
The presence of ≥ 2 of 4 high-yield criteria is 87% sensitive in detecting > 5% dehydration. *Acad Emerg Med 1996;395*	• Capillary refill > 2 seconds • Dry mucous membranes • Absent tears • General ill appearance

IV Maintenance Fluid Calculations

By Body Weight	4 ml/kg/hour (100 ml/kg/day) for 1st 10 kg, + 2 ml/kg/hour (50 ml/kg/day) for 2nd 10 kg, + 1 ml/kg/hour (20 ml/kg/day) for each kg above 20 kg
By Surface Area	Maintenance fluids by BSA (body surface area) = 2,000 ml/m²/day. Normal BSA = square root of [height(cm) x weight (kg) / 3600]

Maintenance Na⁺ requirements = 2-3 mEq/100 ml maintenance fluid administered
Maintenance K⁺ requirements = 2 mEq/100 ml maintenance fluid administered

Composition of Oral and Intravenous Solutions

Solution	Sodium (mEq/l)	Potassium (mEq/l)	Chloride (mEq/l)	Bicarbonate (mEq/l)[1]	Glucose (g/dl)
Extracellular fluid	142	4	103	27	~0.1
0.9NS	154	0	154	0	0
D5NS	154	0	154	0	5
Normosol R	140	5	98	0	0
Plasmalyte	140	10	103	0	0
5% albumin	130-160	0	130-160	0	0
Hypertonic 3%NS	513	0	513	0	0
0.45 NS	77	0	77	0	0
0.3NS	51	0	51	0	0
0.2NS	34	0	34	0	0
LR	130	0	109	28	0
Infant Carvajal's[2]	81	0	61	20	4.65
Child Carvajal's[2]	132	3.8	109	27	4.8
WHO solution[3]	90	20	80	-	2.0
Lytren	50	25	45	30	2.0
Pedialyte	45	20	35	30	2.5
Rehydralyte	75	20	65	30	2.5
Resol	50	20	50	34	2.0
Ricelyte	50	25	45	10	3.0
Infalyte	50	20	40	-	2.0
Gatorade	28	2	-	-	2.1
Ginger ale	4	0.2	-	-	9.0
Coke/Pepsi	3/2	0.1/0.9	13.4/7.3	10.0/10.0	10.5/10.5
Apple/Grape juice	1-4	15-30	-	-	12.0/15.0
Jello	24	1.5	-	-	15.8

1 Or citrate or lactate. [2]Used for burns and contains 12.5 g/L albumin.
3 Excess WHO (World Health Organization) formula causes ↑Na, give with free water.

Oral Rehydration	WHO Recommendations
Wheat and rice-based oral electrolyte solutions are superior to glucose solutions for rehydration, ↓ stool frequency volume.	• 1st hydrate with 100 ml/kg WHO formula over 4 h • Then 50 ml/kg of water or breast milk over next 2h • If still dehydrated, 50 ml/kg WHO formula next 6h • Then 100 ml/kg of WHO formula over next 24 h, then 150 ml/kg/day of WHO formula. Give additional free H₂0 with WHO formula or hypernatremia may occur

Gastrointestinal Disorders

Common GI Therapeutic Agents

Drug	Available forms	Dosing
bisacodyl (*Dulcolax*)	Enema: 10mg/30ml Supp: 5,10 mg Tab: 5 mg	Oral: 5 mg/dose Rectal (≤ 2 years): 5 mg/dose Rectal (> 2 years): 5-10 mg/dose
cimetidine (*Tagamet*)	Injectable: 150 mg/5ml Susp: 300 mg/5ml Tabs: 200,300,400 mg	Neonate: 5-10 mg/kg/day (bid-qid) Infant: 10-20 mg/kg/day (bid - qid) Child: 20-40 mg/kg/day (qid)
docusate Na⁺ (*Colace, DSS*)	Syrup:50 or 60 mg/15ml Solution: 10&50 mg/1ml Tab/Caps: 50,100,250	< 3 years: 10-40 mg (qd-qid) 3-6 years: 20-60 mg (qd-qid) 6-12 years: 40-150 mg (qd-qid)
famotidine (*Pepcid*)	Liquid: 40 mg/5 ml Cap/Tab: 10, 20, 40 mg	0.5-1 mg/kg/day (bid-qhs) Max dose 40 mg/day
glycerin	infant suppository	insert + retain > 5 min (bid or qd prn)
Magic mouth-wash-gingivo-stomatitis	Susp: Add *Benadryl* 30 mg + *Mylanta* 60 ml + *Carafate* 4 g	Apply small amounts to affected area prn or swish and spit. Do not exceed 5 mg/kg of *Benadryl* per day.
metoclopro-mide (*Reglan*)	Injectable: 5 mg/1ml Syrup: 5 mg/5 ml Tabs: 5,10 mg	Reflux: 0.4-0.8 mg/kg/day (qid) Max dose 15 mg
ondansetron (*Zofran*)	Injectable: 2 mg/ml or 32 mg/50 ml Oral Solution: 4 mg/5 ml Tablet: 4, 8, 24	0.1-0.15 mg/kg IV (max 4 mg) 1.6 mg (6-12 mo) PO, 3.2 mg (1-3 y) PO, 4 mg (4-11 y) PO tid q 8h > 11 years: 8 mg PO tid or 24 mg qhs
phosphorolated carbohydrates	(*Emetrol* non-absorbed compound)	5-10 ml PO qid prn
polyethylene glycol(*Miralax*)	PEG 14 oz or 27 oz	25-40 ml/kg/hour until rectal effluent clear. Fast 2 h pre-bowel cleansing
promethazine (*Phenergan*)	Supp: 12.5, 25, 50 mg Syrup: 6.25 mg/5ml Tabs: 12.5, 25, 50 mg	0.25-1.0 mg/kg/dose (q4-6h) (Max dose 25 mg) **CAUTION (may mask serious illness)** use sparingly & > 2 y)
ranitidine (*Zantac*)	Syrup: 15 mg/ml Tabs: 75, 150, 300 mg	Ulcer: 2-4 mg/kg/day (bid/[q4-6h if IV]) GERD/esophagitis: 4-10 mg/kg/day (bid if PO or q 4-6h if IV dosing)
senna (*Senokot*)	Syrup: 218 mg/5 ml Tabs:187, 217, 600	10-20 mg/kg/dose (qhs) If > 27 kg may use ½ supp. qhs
simethicone (*Mylicon, GasX*)	Susp: 40 mg/0.6 ml Tab: 80,125,150,166mg	< 2 years (y) - 20 mg qid; 2-12 y – 40 mg qid, > 12 y – 40-125 mg ac & qhs
sucralfate (*Carafate*)	Susp: 1g/10 ml Tab: 1g	40-80 mg/kg/day (qid); stomatitis – 5-10 ml swish & spit or swallow qid
trimethobenz-amide (*Tigan*)	Supp: 100, 200 Caps: 100, 250	≥ 15 kg: 100-200 mg/dose tid-qid **See promethazine cautions**.

Constipation

Organic Causes of Chronic Constipation	
Endocrine/Metabolic	Congenital pseudo-obstruction, amyloidosis, scleroderma, lupus, diabetes, hypothyroid, hyperparathyroidism, pheochromocytoma, porphyria, graft vs. host disease
Medicines/Drugs	Laxative abuse, diuretics, tricyclic antidepressants, narcotics, aluminum antacids, vincristine, calcium channel blockers, iron ingestion, lead poisoning
Neurologic	Hirschsprung's, neuronal dysplasia, hypoganglionosis, dysautonomia, spinal cord dysplasia/hypotonia syndromes, botulism
Obstructive	Anterior ectopic anus, congenital/acquired anal ring stenosis, small left colon, meconium ileus (cystic fibrosis), strictures (post-surgery or post-NEC), pelvic/abd. mass, pregnancy

Consider above if failure to thrive, pilonidal dimples/hair tuft, sacral agenesis, flat buttocks, anteriorly displaced anus, tight empty rectum with palpable abdominal fecal mass, gush of liquid stool and air from rectum after digital exam, occult blood, absent anal wink, absent cremasteric reflex, or decreased low extremity tone/strength/relaxation phase of DTRs.

Diagnosis/Management Idiopathic Constipation/Soiling in Children

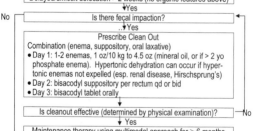

Delayed/difficult defecation > 2 weeks (no organic features above)
↓Yes

No ← Is there fecal impaction?
↓Yes

Prescribe Clean Out
Combination (enema, suppository, oral laxative)
- Day 1: 1-2 enemas, 1 oz/10 kg to 4.5 oz (mineral oil, or if > 2 yo phosphate enema). Hypertonic dehydration can occur if hypertonic enemas not expelled (esp. renal disease, Hirschsprung's)
- Day 2: bisacodyl suppository per rectum qd or bid
- Day 3: bisacodyl tablet orally

Is cleanout effective (determined by physical examination)? → No
↓ Yes

Maintenance therapy using multimodal approach for ≥ 6 months
- Behavior - (sit 4X/day X 10-15 min), document stool passage
- Diet (> 1 year) – fiber intake of (age + 5) grams/day, ensure adequate fluids, restrict constipating foods
- Meds (> 6 months) – mineral oil, magnesium salts or lactulose 1-3 ml/kg/day, OR senna 5 ml/day if 1-5 y, 10 ml/day if > 5 y
- Structured follow up to ensure compliance
- Wean from laxatives after 6 months and end full maintenance
- Reconsider organic cause if < 3 stool/week or soiling at 6 mo.

Arch Pediatr Adolesc Med 1999; 153: 380.

Diarrhea

Secretory diarrhea is enterotoxin-induced, (e.g., E coli, vibrio, clostridia, some staphylococcal species, shigella, salmonella). Enterotoxins cause fluid and electrolyte secretion from crypt cells and block absorption of Na^+ and Cl^- by the carrier mechanism. Glucose coupled Na^+ absorption is not blocked. Fecal Na^+ is > 60 mosm/L and stool osmotic gap [290 – 2X(stool Na^+ + stool K^+)] < 100 mOsm/L.

Cytotoxic diarrhea is usually due to viral agents (e.g., rotavirus) and is characterized by destruction of villous mucosa. Shortened villi decrease the intestinal surface area available for fluid absorption.

Osmotic diarrhea is usually due to malabsorption syndromes (e.g., lactose intolerance). Osmotically active agents retain fluid in the bowel lumen. Osmotic diarrhea exacerbates cytotoxic and secretory diarrhea through impaired absorption of nutrients and electrolytes. Orally administered magnesium sulfate and sorbitol cause osmotic diarrhea. Fecal Na^+ is < 70 mosm/L and stool osmotic gap [290 – 2X(stool Na^+ + stool K^+)] > 100 mOsm/L. Fecal pH < 5.5 or stool reducing substances > 0.25-0.5% suggests carbohydrate malabsorption.

Dysenteric diarrhea is due to invasion of mucosa and submucosa of the colon and terminal ileum by infectious agents (e.g., salmonella, shigella, yersinia, campylobacter, enteroviruses). Edema, bleeding, and leukocyte infiltration typically occur.

Clinical Evaluation of the Child with Diarrhea

Rotavirus is the most common etiology of infectious diarrhea. A bacterial origin is associated with blood in the stool in 50% of cases, and neutrophils in the stool in 70% of cases. Fecal pH < 5.5 or stool reducing substances > 0.25-0.5% suggests carbohydrate malabsorption. Bacterial diarrheas are more common in summer. Day care centers are associated with shigella, giardia, and rotavirus. Other etiologies for diarrhea include antibiotics, intussusception, gastrointestinal bleeding, and hemolytic-uremic syndrome.

Diarrhea Therapy

See page 56 for American Academy of Pediatric Guidelines for Managing Acute Gastroenteritis. Oral Rehydration Therapy (ORT) is often effective, as co-transport of sodium with glucose remains intact in all types of diarrhea. World Health Organization (WHO) solution can be used in all ages (including neonates) and in those with hypotonic, isotonic, or hypertonic dehydration.

In hypernatremia, oral therapy may be superior to IV therapy. Standard glucose electrolyte solutions (e.g., *Pedialyte, Lytren*) supply electrolytes and water to correct dehydration but do not decrease stool output and have no nutritional value. Rice and wheat-based ORT are superior to standard ORT in correcting rehydration and decreasing stool output. Some clear liquids such as juices, sodas, and jello are inappropriate for treating acute diarrhea, as they contain little sodium and have high carbohydrate content which increases the osmotic load and may aggravate diarrhea (especially apple juice).

Refeeding: Gut rest is not useful. Early feeding hastens mucosal recovery and shortens the duration of illness despite increasing stool output. Breast feeding is well-tolerated. Full strength feeds are best. Some children with prolonged diarrhea develop lactose intolerance, but the majority tolerate lactose well. A BRAT diet along with wheat noodles and potatoes can be started at once. High-starch and low-fat foods are generally helpful.

Drug Therapy: Kaolin-pectin (*Kaopectate*) is an absorbent. Bismuth subsalicylate (*PeptoBismol*) inhibits intestinal secretions and is useful in traveler's diarrhea. Antibiotics are indicated for shigella, vibrio cholera, and enteroinvasive E coli. Sulfamethoxazole/trimethoprim (*Septra* or *Bactrim*) is the drug of choice for shigella, vibrio, and E coli. Antibiotics for salmonella are indicated if < 3-6 months old, toxic, or immunocompromised. Erythromycin is effective for campylobacter. See pages 77-83 for antibiotic recommendations and dosing for specific organisms.

Chronic diarrhea: Culture the stool and test for lactose intolerance (reducing substances > 0.25-0.5% and pH < 5.5). If lactose intolerance suspected, discontinue dairy products for 2 weeks.

Discharge instructions for diarrhea
- Administer clear liquids such as *Pedialyte, Lytren*, and *Ricelyte* in smaller children. Older children may be given *Powerade* or *Gatorade*. Do not give plain water or juices. If no vomiting, administer large amounts of fluid every 3-4 hours. If vomiting, give small sips every 10-15 minutes; slowly increase amount and decrease frequency of feeding.
- Start refeeding in 8 to 24 hours even if diarrhea is present. In an infant, start with full-strength regular formula. If the diarrhea is prolonged or worsens after administration of lactose-based formula switch to a soy-based formula.
- If child tolerates solids, give a BRAT diet (bananas, rice, applesauce, toast) and noodles or potatoes.
- Physician reevaluation if bloody stool, bilious vomiting, or worsened symptoms.

American Academy of Pediatrics
Practice Guideline for Managing Acute Gastroenteritis

Obtain History & Perform Physical Examination
(1 month-5 year old with diarrhea)

↓

Obtain current weight OR
Estimate % dehydration (see page 50)

↓

Is one of following present
• ≥ 10% dehydration
• shock or altered mental status
• ileus

→ YES → • 20-40 ml/kg NS or LR IV X 1 hour
• Repeat if needed
• Begin oral hydration
• Hospitalize

↓ NO

6-9% dehydrated by
weight loss or clinical
estimate (page 50)

→ YES → Oral rehydration at 100
ml/kg over 4 hours PLUS
replace ongoing loss

↓ NO

3-5% dehydrated by
weight loss or clinical
estimate (page 50)

→ YES → Oral rehydration at 50 ml/kg
over 4 hours PLUS replace
ongoing loss

↓ NO

< 3% dehydrated by
weight loss or clinical
estimate (page 50)

Is patient tolerating
oral therapy?

→ YES → Continue oral
therapy for 4-6
hours or until
rehydrated

↓ NO

Continue regular diet
Consider added
glucose electrolyte

Begin IV therapy
Consider NG tube

Resume breast
feed, formula, milk,
regular foods, &
replace ongoing
loss with glucose
electrolyte solution

A double blind placebo controlled study found that
administration of ondansetron (*Zofran*) 1.6 mg (6-12
mo), 3.2 mg (1-3 y), 4 mg (4-12 y) PO q 8 h X 6 doses
led to ↓ vomiting, IV fluid use, and admission rates.
[4mg/5ml sol'n]   *Ann Emerg Med* 2002; 39: 397.

Specific AAP recommendations:
• Use oral rehydration therapy for mild to moderate dehydration
• Children who require rehydration should continue to be fed age appropriate
  diets after rehydration (early feeding will decrease duration of diarrhea)
• As a general rule, pharmacologic agents should not be used for acute diarrhea
  (opiates/atropine are contraindicated, anticholinergic agents/Bismuth
  subsalicylate, adsorbents, lactobacillus compounds are not recommended)

AAP. *Pediatrics* 1996; 97: 424.

Upper Gastrointestinal Bleeding - Etiology

Age	Most Frequent Cause	Features
0-30 days	• Ingested maternal blood • Bleeding diathesis • Gastric ulcers • Gastritis, esophagitis	See Apt Downey test See below[1] Premature, other stressors
> 30 days – 2 years	• Stress ulcers • Gastritis, esophagitis, Mallory Weiss tears (MW)	
2-6 years	• Gastric ulcer, gastritis, varices • Esophagitis, MW, hemophilia	
> 6 years	• Peptic ulcer, gastritis • Esophagitis	Reflux, chemical, infection

[1] Hemorrhagic disease newborn, aspirin, phenytoin, phenobarb., promethazine

Most Common Causes of Lower GI bleed Presenting to a Pediatric ED

Age	Etiology	%
< 1 month	• Allergic colitis (allergy to milk/soy protein) • Anorectal fissure • Vaginal bleeding • Other causes (maternal blood [see Apt-Downey test – page 58], bleeding diathesis, infectious, necrotizing enterocolitis, volvulus,Hirschprung's)	69% 15% 8% -
1-12 months	• Anorectal fissure • Allergic colitis • Infectious • Unknown lower source • Intussusception (see page 137) • Other causes (lymphoid nodular hyperplasia, - Meckel's, juvenile polyps, intestinal duplication, hemolytic uremic syndrome – see page 65)	27% 23% 19% 15% 12% -
1-5 years	• Unknown lower (or upper GI) source • Red food ingestion, infectious • Anorectal fissure • Chemotherapy, foreign body, ulcer,colon polyp • Other causes (Juvenile polyps, intussusception page 137, Meckel's, inflammatory bowel, Henoch Schonlein Purpura – page 65)	29% 19% each 14% 5% each -
5 years *Ann Emerg Med* 1994; 23: 1253.	• Unknown lower source • Infectious • Anorectal fissure • Rectal varices, Inflammatory bowel disease • Red food ingestion • Hemorrhoids, chemotherapy, Meckel's, colon polyp, lymphoid nodular hyperplasia	29% 20% 14% 9% each 6% 3% each

Evaluation and Management of GI Bleeding

- Place cardiac monitor, administer O_2, and insert two large bore IV's.
- Draw CBC, clotting studies, type and cross at least 15 ml/kg of packed RBC's.
- Administer 20 ml/kg NS bolus and repeat to correct hypotension or shock.
- Consider blood transfusion if there is no response to first two fluid boluses.
- **Pharmacotherapy** - For variceal bleeding in addition to above consider vasopressin (0.002-0.005 U/kg/minute, titrate to maximum of 0.01 U/kg/min) or octreotide [*Sandostatin*] (1-5 µg/kg IV or SC q 12 h). Multiple serious side effects can occur with either medication; therefore, intensive monitoring is required if either is administered.
- **Endoscopy** identifies bleeding site in 75-90% of upper GI bleeding and can be used to coagulate or sclerose upper GI bleeding site.
- **Urgent surgery** indications: unrelenting hemorrhage, > 50-75 ml/kg blood transfused in 2 hours, perforation, or vascular compromise.
- **Contrast studies** are not indicated acutely. Angiography will only detect a bleeding site if the bleeding rate is > 0.5-2.0 ml/minute.
- **Radionuclide scanning** (Tc99) may detect low grade GI bleeding from a Meckel's diverticulum. Tc99 has an affinity for parietal cells present in gastric mucosa and in 90% of Meckel's diverticulum. A positive scan consists of a persistent focus of uptake in the right lower quadrant or lower abdomen. This test is indicated for any child < 3 years old who presents with painless lower GI bleeding. This test is 85% sensitive and 92% specific for Meckel's.

Erroneous Stool Guaiac Testing: Acidic pH lowers the sensitivity of guaiac, so use specific gastric test cards (e.g., *Gastroccult*) when evaluating blood from an upper gastrointestinal source.

- *False positive:* Iron, red fruits, meats, iodine, bromide, horseradish, turnips, tomatoes, fresh red cherries or chlorophyll
- *False negative:* Dried stool specimens, outdated reagent or guaiac card, bile, vitamin C or certain antacids

Apt-Downey Test for Fetal vs. Maternal Blood: Mix stool in a test tube with an equal quantity of tap water. Centrifuge or filter out solids. Add one part 1.0% NaOH to five parts of supernatant. Read in 2 minutes. Fetal Hb resists alkali denaturation. A persistent pink color indicates the presence of fetal Hb. If supernatant turns yellow, Hb is adult and thus maternal.

Neonatal - Jaundice

Newborns exhibit hepatic insufficiency that resolves in 1st 4-6 weeks. 50th percentile for bilirubin in normal neonates is 6 mg/dl (6% have levels > 12 mg/dl) Jaundice is usually noted at 5 mg/dl in infants & 2 mg/dl if older. Hyperbilirubinemia is associated with breast feeding, weight loss, maternal diabetes, Asian ethnicity, oxytocin, ↓gestational age, & male sex. Prolonged unconjugated hyperbilirubinemia can lead to kernicterus. Precise level of bilirubin that is toxic for an individual infant is unknown. Early signs of kernicterus: lethargy, poor feeding, loss of Moro reflex, seizures and movement disorders (late sign). Direct bilirubin should be ≤ 15% of total (conjugated + unconjugated or direct + indirect). Conjugated hyperbilirubinemia is abnormal and should always provoke further evaluation.

Hyperbilirubinemia Management for Healthy Term Newborns

Age *(if < 24 hours old see below)*	25-48 hrs	49-72 hrs	> 72 hrs
	Total serum bilirubin in mg/dl (µmol/L)		
Consider Phototherapy	≥ 12 (170)	≥ 15 (260)	≥ 17 (290)
Phototherapy	≥ 15 (260)	≥ 18 (310)	≥ 20 (340)
Exchange Therapy if Phototherapy Fails	≥ 20 (340)	≥ 25 (430)	≥ 25 (430)
Exchange Therapy and Phototherapy	≥ 25 (430)	≥ 30 (510)	≥ 30 (510)

Pediatrics 1994;565

Factors Associated with Non-physiologic Jaundice

- Jaundice in infant < 24 hours old or non-breastfed infant > 1 week old
- Serum bilirubin rise of > 5 mg/dl/day or > 0.5 mg/dl/hour
- Serum bilirubin > 15 mg/dl in a full term neonate (lower if premature)
- Jaundice persisting > 1 week in a full term or more than 2 weeks if postterm
- Conjugated ↑ bili (e.g., obstruction, infection, toxin/drugs or metabolic/genetic)
- Ill appearance, infection or GI obstruction suspected, or abnormal labs below

Evaluation of Neonatal Jaundice

All patients	total bilirubin, look up maternal Rh
Additional tests (depending on age, presentation)	Direct/indirect bilirubin, CBC, manual differential, reticulocyte count & peripheral smear, blood type and Rh analysis, Coomb's test (esp. if mother's blood type unknown)
If >1 week old add	Liver and thyroid function tests
Consider	Work-ups for sepsis & TORCH, evaluation for GI obstruction

Treatment of Hyperbilirubinemia

- Exchange transfusion if bilirubin > 20-25 mg/dl in a term neonate, or lower level in premature neonate (exact level controversial)
- Phototherapy if within 5 mg/dl of exchange transfusion level
- Phototherapy if there is an ↑ total serum bilirubin of > 1-2 mg/dl in 4-6 hours
- Perform exchange transfusion at lower levels if signs of kernicterus are present
- Treat underlying disorder (e.g. sepsis, GI tract obstruction)

Anemia

Normal RBC Indices (mean ± 2 standard deviations)

Age	Hb(g/dl)	Hct(%)	MCV(fl)	MCH(pg)	MCHC(g/dl)
Birth	16.5 ± 3.0	51 ± 9	108 ± 10	34 ± 3	33 ± 3
1-3 days	18.5 ± 4.0	56 ± 14	108 ± 13	34 ± 3	33 ± 4
1 week	17.5 ± 4.0	54 ± 12	107 ± 19	34 ± 6	33 ± 5
2 weeks	16.5 ± 4.0	51 ± 12	105 ± 19	34 ± 6	33 ± 5
1 month	14.0 ± 4.0	43 ± 12	104 ± 19	34 ± 6	33 ± 5
2 months	11.5 ± 2.5	35 ± 7	96 ± 19	30 ± 4	33 ± 4
3-6 months	11.5 ± 2.0	35 ± 6	91 ± 17	30 ± 5	33 ± 3
0.5-2 years	12.0 ± 1.5	36 ± 3	78 ± 8	27 ± 4	33 ± 3
2-6 years	12.5 ± 1.0	37 ± 3	81 ± 6	27 ± 3	34 ± 3
6-12 years	13.5 ± 2.0	40 ± 5	86 ± 9	29 ± 4	34 ± 3
12-18y female	14.0 ± 2.0	41 ± 5	90 ± 12	30 ± 5	34 ± 3
12-18y male	14.5 ± 1.5	43 ± 6	88 ± 10	30 ± 5	34 ± 3

Causes of Anemia by Age

Neonate: Blood loss, isoimmunization or congenital hemolytic anemia
3-6 months: Congenital disorder of hemoglobin synthesis (e.g., thalassemia)
6 months to 2 years: Iron deficiency is associated with early or excessive cow's milk. Hereditary hemolytic anemia (spherocytosis, hemoglobinopathy, or red cell enzyme deficiency) suggested by a family history of anemia, jaundice, gallstones or splenectomy. B_{12} deficiency suggested by tortuous retinal vessels (hemoglobinopathy), glossitis and diminished vibratory/position sense. RBC distribution width (RDW) reflects cell heterogeneity. Variable RDW sizes are seen in hemolysis or reticulocytosis. Markedly high WBC counts, high glucose, sodium, and triglycerides falsely elevate RBC counts.

Anemia Differential Diagnosis

Microcytic	Iron deficiency (RDW > 14%), thalassemia (RDW < 14%), chronic inflammation, sideroblastic anemia, lead poisoning, B_6 deficiency
Macrocytic	Folic acid or B_{12} deficiency, Fanconi's, hepatic disease
Normocytic (high retics)	*Extrinsic disorders*: antibody-mediated hemolysis, fragmentation hemolysis, DIC, hemolytic uremic syndrome, artificial heart valves, liver and renal disease. *Intrinsic disorders*: membrane disorders (spherocytosis, elliptocytosis), enzyme deficiencies (glucose-6-phosphate dehydrogenase or pyruvate kinase deficiency), hemoglobin disorders (SS, SC, S-thalassemia)
Normocytic (low retics)	Diamond Blackfan, transient erythroblastopenia of childhood, aplastic crisis, bone marrow infiltrate (leukemia, metastatic disease), renal disease, infection, malnutrition

Sickle Cell Anemia

Diagnosis and evaluation of patients with sickle cell disease

- Sickle cell screen may be negative up to 4-6 months of age and in sickle trait.
- A routine Hb is recommended to assess severity or change of anemia.
- Consider a reticulocyte count to screen for aplastic crisis (Mean reticulocyte for sickle cell patient is 12%, in aplastic crises it may be <3%).
- Urine specific gravity is not a useful test for dehydration, as it may be low from isosthenuria (inability to concentrate the urine).
- Profound and sudden decrease in Hb combined with increased reticulocyte count is suggestive of splenic sequestration crisis (see below)

Fever in Sickle Cell Anemia

Penicillin prophylaxis decreases the incidence of sepsis and death for sickle cell children aged 6 months to 5 years. As a rule, febrile children with sickle cell disease are admitted and treated with IV antibiotics. However, criteria have been published that define a subset of patients that may be treated as outpatients.

Criteria for Outpatient Management of Fever in Sickle Cell Patients

• Yale observation score < 10 (pg 88)	• WBC count > 5,000 and < 30,000
• Normal blood pressure	• Hb > 5 g/dl, Platelets > 100,000
• No prior pneumococcal sepsis	• Administer ceftriaxone 50 mg/kg
• Mild pain only	IV/IM if no allergy to cephalosporin
• No pneumonia	• Reliable 24 hour follow up with
• Normal capillary refill	repeat ceftriaxone dose in 24 hours
• Temperature < 40°C (104°F)	

Wilimas. *New Engl J Med* 1993; 329: 472

Management of Sickle Cell Disease Complications

Painful crises (all ages) Most common sites of pain in order of decreasing frequency: lumbosacral spine, thigh and hip, knee, abdomen, shoulder, chest. Intravenous morphine is the treatment of choice, and should be titrated. Meperidine is not recommended (especially in high or repeated doses), as a metabolite (normeperidine) can cause CNS excitation and seizures. Hydration (oral or IV) and oxygen are commonly accepted adjuncts.

Splenic sequestration crisis (1 - 6 years) Associated with an acute drop of Hb >3 g/dl or total Hb <6 g/dl. Due to splenic vein vaso-occlusion. Abdominal pain, shock, and hypotension may occur. Second only to sepsis as cause of death in children with sickle cell. Patients are usually < 6 years old if SS disease (functional asplenia) but older if SC or S-B-thalassemia variants. Patients present with sudden hypovolemic shock or a slow increase in spleen size. Obtain CBC, type and cross, and reticulocyte count. Admit and treat hypovolemia.

Management of Sickle Cell Disease Complications

Acute chest syndrome (all ages) Defined as complex of pulmonary symptoms and a pulmonary infiltrate in a patient with sickle cell disease. Admit and treat as sickle crisis, with oxygen, fluids, transfusion prn, empiric antibiotics (e.g., erythromycin and cefuroxime).

Hand foot syndrome (dactylitis, 6 months to 6 years) Due to vaso-occlusion in the hands and feet. This syndrome is the most common presentation of sickle cell anemia at 6-24 months, and often the first crisis experienced. Nonpitting edema from symmetric infarction of the metacarpals/metatarsals occurs. Treat as a pain crisis.

Sickle stroke (all ages) Occurs in 10-20% of children with sickle cell disease. Mean age is 10 years. Strokes are usually ischemic, although hemorrhagic strokes may occur in older children. Treat by exchange transfusion to keep hemoglobin S < 20% of total.

Aplastic crisis (6 months to young adulthood) Parvovirus is the most common identified precipitant. Other common causes include drug toxicity (phenylbutazone) and folate deficiency. Hallmark is reticulocyte count < 3%. Transfuse these patients if they are severely anemic.

Cardiac complications Patients may develop congestive heart failure.

Abdominal complications Liver, splenic and mesenteric infarctions may occur. Bilirubin gallstones are common although < 10% are symptomatic.

Genitourinary complications Priapism may develop. Priapism lasting > 3 hours is unlikely to resolve spontaneously. Treatment of priapism consists of hydration, oxygen, pain management, and possibly exchange transfusion. These patients are less likely to require surgery to correct priapism than patients without sickle cell disease. Additionally, painless hematuria and renal papillary necrosis may occur, and isosthenuria (difficulty concentrating urine) may develop.

Bone complications Avascular necrosis of the femoral head occurs in 12% of patients. Sickle dactylitis can cause small lytic lesions in the digits.

Causes of Abnormal Bleeding Tests[1]

Lab Value	Causes
thrombocytopenia ↓platelet count (<150,000/ml)	Decreased production of platelets (due to drugs, toxins or infections), splenic sequestration or platelet pooling, platelet destruction (due to collagen vascular disease, drugs, post transfusion, infection, ITP, DIC, TTP, HUS, or vasculitis)
platelet dysfunction (with normal count)	Adhesion defects (e.g., von Willibrand's disease) or aggregation defects (e.g., thrombasthenia)
↑BT (>9 minutes)	All platelet disorders, DIC, ITP, uremia, liver failure, aspirin
↑PTT (>35 sec)	Coagulation pathway defects (common factors 2, 5, 10, intrinsic 8, 9, 11, 12, von Willibrand's), DIC, liver failure, heparin
↑PT (>12-13 sec)	Coagulation pathway defects (common factors 2, 5, 10, extrinsic 7) DIC, liver failure, warfarin
↑TT (>8-10 sec)	DIC, liver failure or uremia, heparin
↓ fibrinogen, ↑FSP	ITP, liver failure

[1] BT-bleeding time, TT-Thrombin time, PTT-partial thromboplastin time, PT-prothrombin time, DIC-disseminated intravascular coagulopathy, ITP-idiopathic thrombocytopenic purpura, TTP-thrombotic thrombocytopenic purpura, HUS-hemolytic uremic syndrome.

Platelet and capillary disorders cause mucous membrane bleeds (GI, epistaxis, prolonged bleed with cuts, petechiae (↑bleeding time and abnormal platelets).
Coagulation disorders cause deep muscle, CNS bleeds, hemarthrosis, ↑PT/PTT.

Dosing of Replacement Factors

Medication	Dose
Factor VIII	• [desired activity level (%) – baseline activity level (%)] ÷2 • 1 unit/kg factor 8↑activity level 2% (factor 8 T½ = 12 hours)[1]
Factor IX	• desired activity level (%) - baseline activity level (%) • 1 unit/kg factor 9↑activity level 1% (factor 9 T½ = 24 hours) [1]
DDAVP *Desmopressin*	• 0.3 µg/kg in 50 ml NS IV over 30 minutes • possibly effective via nasal spray or SC injection, recommended only if baseline activity > 10%

[1] T½ = half life

Factor Replacements

Product	Forms	Contents	Units/bag[1]
cryoprecipitate	cryoprecipitate	factor VII, vWf [2] fibrinogen,	100
factor VIII	*Recombinate, Bioclate, Kogenate* (all recombinant factor 8)	factor VIII, human albumin	250,500, 1000
factor IX	*Konyne, Feiba, Alphanine, Proplex, Autoplex,* prothrombin concentrates	factors II, VIII, IX, X	400-600

[1] Units/bag should be indicated on the label. [2]von Willebrand factor

Factor VIII Deficiency Treatment

Bleed type	%Activity Desired	Dose[1] (units/kg)	Duration of Therapy
Severe[1]			
CNS injury	80-100%	50	14 days
GI bleed	80-100%	50	3 days more than bleed
Major trauma	80-100%	50	depends on injuries
Retroperitoneal	80-100%	50	6 days
Retropharyngeal	80-100%	50	4 days
Pending surgery	80-100%	50	variable
Moderate[2]			
Mild head trauma	50%	25	variable
Deep muscle	50%	25	q day until resolution
Hip or groin injury	40%	20	repeat once in 1-2 days
Mouth, lip, dental[3]	40%	20	variable
Hematuria[4]	40%	20	3-5 days
Mild[2]			
Laceration[5]	20%	10	until sutures out for 24h
Common joint	20-40%	10-20	recheck in 1-2 days
Soft tissue / Small muscle[6]	20-40%	10-20	variable

[1] If baseline activity is 0%. Assume all severe bleeding cases have baseline of 0%.

[2] Desmopressin (DDAVP) 0.3 μg/kg IV or intranasal or subcutaneous has been used for mild and moderate bleeding states, especially useful if baseline factor is > 10%.

[3] To prepare for dental/oropharyngeal procedures, consider aminocaproic acid (*Amicar*) 100 mg/kg PO q6h for 6 days or cyclokapron 25 mg/kg q6h for 6 days. Also consider topical epinephrine, *Surgicel*, or *Avitene*. CAUTERY MAY WORSEN BLEEDING.

[4] Consider prednisone (2 mg/kg/day x 2d) and oral fluids without factor replacement if mild.

[5] Epistaxis and minor lacerations may not need replacement.

[6] Consider admission to observe for compartment syndrome.

Other Treatment Options in Hemophilia

Inhibitors: Patients with inhibitors may have poor response to factor VIII. Factor VIII may be used to treat if low titer inhibitor (<2 Bethesda Unit Titer [BUT]) or Factor IX at 50-100 units/kg if minor bleeds. If significant bleed, use ↑ doses of factor VIII. If high titer of inhibitor (>10 BUT) and activated factor IX concentrates are not successful ± plasmaphoresis and factor replacement or porcine factor concentrate.

Fresh frozen plasma (FFP) contains all coagulation factors and used for unknown bleeding disorders. FFP or cryoprecipitate can be used to treat von Willebrand's. FFP 40 ml/kg raises activity of any factor to 100%. May cause fluid overload.

Cryoprecipitate - 5-10 U factor 8 activity/ml (1bag = 10ml, 50-100U factor 8 activity).

Desmopressin (DDAVP) - 0.3 μg/kg in NS IV over 30 min. Mild to moderate bleeding in von Willebrand's & hemophilia A. Causes seizures/↓Na < 4 yo.

Prothrombin complex (factors 2, 7, 9, 10) can be used to treat hemophilia B but can precipitate thrombi and/or disseminated intravascular coagulation (DIC).

Hemolytic Uremic Syndrome (HUS)

HUS - a post-infectious disorder causing (1) nephropathy, (2) microangiopathic hemolytic anemia, & (3) thrombocytopenia. It commonly occurs < 5 years old following a URI or gastroenteritis (esp. E. coli 0157:H7, *Shigella, Salmonella*). Organisms pro-duce toxin that kills GI organ cells. 30% reoccur. **Treatment:** Manage complications: dialysis (acute renal failure), anti-hypertensives (if↑BP), fluids & blood (bleed or↓BP), anti-seizure medications prn, platelets prn. *Dialyze* if (1) congestive heart failure (2) BUN > 100 mg/dl, (3) encephalopathy, (4) anuria > 24 hours (5) ↑K⁺

Clinical Features
• *Prodome* - URI or gastroenteritis
• *GI* – 75% have pain (can cause intussusception, or perforation), vomiting, or diarrhea (often bloody)
• ↓*Urination* (gross hematuria rare)
• *Skin* – pallor, petechiae, purpura
• *Hypertension* (in up to 50%)
• *CNS*- seizure, coma, encephalopathy

Laboratory Features
• Urine – hematuria, proteinuria, casts
• CBC – ↓Hb, ↓ platelets, ↓WBC
• Smear – schistocytes, helmet cells
• ↓Na⁺,↓CO₂,↑K⁺,↑BUN,↑creatinine
• PT/PTT are usually normal

Henoch-Schonlein Purpura

Overview HSP is a systemic vasculitis with skin, joint, GI, or renal involvement. Scrotal, CNS, heart, and lung involvement are less common. HSP without skin involvement is called *HSP syndrome*. HSP peaks at 4-5 years, but can occur at any age. It is more common in winter & early spring. Precipitants: streptococci, mycoplasma, hepatitis B, salicylates, antibiotics, and food allergens. HSP is pathophysiologically a small vessel vasculitis, with WBC's infiltrating and necrosing the walls of capillaries, arterioles, and venules. **Treatment** Supportive care and steroids are used for abdominal pain and renal involvement, although their benefit has not been clearly established.

Clinical features
• *Skin* – involved in most. Petechiae, coalesce to large ecchymoses. Purpura are gravity dependent occurring on the buttock and legs.
• *Painful edema* – 25-35% (usually at dorsum of hands and feet), with painful edema of face, scalp.
• *GI tract* – 50-90% with vomiting, or bleeding. Intussusception (3-6%), pancreatitis, or bowel infarcts occur.
• *Joint* involvement in 50-75% usually knees/ankles, transitory periarticular swelling, non-migratory. This is 1ˢᵗ site in 25% & resolves with rest
• *Renal* – 50% and may be the only site that is permanent. Episodic gross hematuria occurs in 30-40%.

Idiopathic Thrombocytopenic Purpura

Overview ITP is an autoimmune disorder with antibodies vs. platelets. ITP is most common platelet disorder in children often between ages of 1 & 4 y. 70% have prior viral infection (e.g. rubella, rubeola). Bone marrow has normal WBCs, & RBCs. Eosinophilia & megakaryocytes (immature/basophilic stippling) may be present.

Treatment may be indicated if bleeding or platelets < 10,000-20,000/mm³. Debate exists as to treatment indications.

Clinical features
• *Skin* – bruising and petechiae are most common
• *Mucous membranes* – epistaxis, gum & GYN bleeding & hematuria are less common than skin manifestations
• *Hematologic* – platelets usually < 20,000/mm³, ± anemia
• *GI* – liver, spleen, and lymph nodes are not enlarged
• *CNS* – most common life threat
• *Systemic* – ± HIV, lupus, lymphoma

Options: (1) prednisone 2 mg/kg/d X 4-8 weeks (2) IV immune globulin 0.8-1.0 g/kg repeat in 24 h if platelets < 40,000, (3) IV anti-D immune globulin 45-50 μg/kg (Ig vs D antigen of RBCs) leads to Hb drop of 0.5-2.0 g/dl. Only effective if Rh positive, (4) plasmapheresis, (5) platelet transfusion of 0.2 U/kg (max 10-12 units) OR 0.4 U/kg IV (max 20 units) if intracranial bleeding (6) splenectomy if persists > 1 year or severe case that does not respond to steroids.

Oncologic Emergencies

Hyperviscosity (Hyperleukocytosis) Syndrome

Etiology	Diagnosis
↑ Serum proteins with sludging & ↓ circulation. Common causes: leukemia (esp. ALL).	• WBC (esp. blasts)>100,000 cells/mm³ • ↑serum viscosity -Ostwald viscometer • Serum protein electrophoresis
Clinical Features	**Management**
• Fatigue, headache, somnolence • Dyspnea, interstitial infiltrates, hypoxia, RV failure, renal failure • ↓ Vision, seizure, deafness, MI • Retinal bleed and exudates	• IV NS, plasmaphoresis • Platelets if count < 20,000/mm³ • Phlebotomy with NS, and exchange transfusion (keep Hb ≤ 10 g/dl) • Anti-leukemic therapy

Massive Hepatomegaly

Clinical Features	Management
• Associated with tumor infiltrate (esp. neuroblastoma & < 4 weeks old) • May cause mechanical compromise of lungs, heart, GI/renal systems, or disseminated intravasc coagulation	• Treat persistent emesis, hypoxia, leg edema, renal insufficiency, or DIC • Chemotherapy • Low dose radiation 150 cGy/day X 3 • Surgical enlargement abdominal wall

Infectious Disease Society Guidelines for Unexplained Fever & Neutropenia

Fever – single oral temp ≥ 38.3°C (101°F) or ≥ 38°C (100.4°F) over at least 1 hour
Neutropenia – neutrophil count < 500/mm³ or< 1,000/mm³ with predicted ≤500/mm³
Evaluation – blood culture (peripheral and catheter), culture lesions, urine and stool, CXR, CBC with diff, liver function tests, electrolytes

---

Antimicrobials for Neutropenia (alternate dosing may be needed if < 3-6 months old)
(1) ceftazidime (*Fortaz*) 150 mg/kg/d (max 12 g/day) IV q 6-8h **OR** (2) imipenem (*Primaxin*) 60-100 mg/kg/day divide q 6 h (max 4 g/day) **OR** (3) cefepime (*Maxipime*) 50 mg/kg (max 2 g/dose) IV q 8 h **OR** (3) aminoglycoside PLUS antipseudomonal β-lactam [*Zosyn, Timentin*] **ADD** vancomycin 10 mg/kg (max 500 mg) IV q 6 h if any of: ↓BP, central catheter, chemotherapy + ↑ mucosal damage, prophylaxis with quinolones before fever, known colonization with pneumococci resistant to penicillin, known gram positive blood culture before susceptibility testing known.

Clin Infect Dis 1997;25:551; J Pediatr 1991; 119: 679.

Spinal Cord Compression

≥ 90% due sarcomas (rhabdo, Ewing's, osteogenic), neuroblastoma, & lymphoma.

Clinical features		*Diagnosis* – plain films are abnormal in only
Back pain	80%	35%, bone scan in 54%. Use CT & MRI instead.
Weakness	67%	*Management* – (1) Dexamethasone 1 mg/kg IV,
Local back tenderness	67%	then 0.25 to 0.5 mg/kg PO q 6 hours, (2)
Paraplegia	57%	surgical decompression [esp. previously
Sphincter dysfunction	57%	unknown tumor type], (3) radiation or
Sensory abnormality	14%	chemotherapy depending on cancer sensitivity

J Neurosurg 1991;74:70; Pediatrics 1986;78:438; Pediatr Clin North Am 1997;44:809.

Superior Vena Cava Syndrome

Anterior > middle mediastinal mass (most common lymphoma, Hodgkins, ALL) or clot (e.g. central venous catheter) obstructing superior vena cava.

Clinical Features – headache, swollen face, altered mental status, syncope dyspnea, plethora, vein distention of face/neck/arms, trachea compressed *Diagnosis* - CXR, CT, MRI. ECG/Echo if ? cardiac & PFTs if pulm. involvement	*Management* • Radiation (can ↑ swelling, cause resp. deterioration, distort histology) • Cyclophosphamide ± vincristine & anthracycline if non-Hodgkins or Hodgkins lymphoma suspected.

Tumor Lysis Syndrome

Occurs within 1-2 days of treatment initiation (esp. leukemias/ALL and lymphomas). *Clinical features* are due to hyperuricemia (renal failure), ↑K⁺ (arrhythmias), ↑phosphate (renal failure), and ↓Ca⁺² (cramping, tetany, confusion, seizures).

Management	*Criteria for Hemodialysis*
• Hydration with NS (no K⁺) ± diuretics	• K⁺ > 6 mEq/L OR Cr > 10 X normal
• Allopurinol 100 mg/m² PO/day	• Uric acid > 10 mg/dl OR P > 10 mg/dl
• Alkalinize serum with NaHCO₃ to urine pH ≥ 7.0 OR *Diamox*	• Symptomatic hypocalcemia
	• Uncontrolled hypertension or uremia

Blood Products and Transfusion (see page 70 for dosing)

Crossmatching and ordering blood products: Type-specific non-crossmatched blood causes a fatality in 1 in 30 million transfusions. Non-ABO antibodies occur in 0.04% of non-transfused and 0.3% of previously transfused.

Whole blood has no WBC's and 20% of normal platelets after 24 h storage. Factors V + VIII decline to 40% after 21 d. 70% of RBC's remain after 21-35 d storage. With storage, K^+ & ammonia increase (beware in liver failure) and Ca^{+2} decreases (beware in liver dysfunction as citrate is not effectively metabolized by the liver).

Packed Red Blood Cells (PRBC's): Hematocrit rises 1% for each ml/kg of PRBC's transfused. Fewer antigens are present in PRBC's compared to whole blood. (1) *Leukocyte poor RBC's* are derived from filtering RBC's and should be used if one (severe), or two (sequential) febrile non-hemolytic transfusion reactions. (2) *Washed RBC's* are useful if prior anaphylaxis due to antibodies to IgA or other proteins. (3) *Frozen deglycerolized RBC's* are the purest RBC product. Use if there is a reaction to washed RBC's or a transfusion reaction due to Anti-IgA antibodies.

Fresh frozen plasma (FFP) ABO cross-match prior to transfusion. Indications: (1) coagulation protein deficiency when specific factor concentrates are undesirable or unavailable, (2) warfarin reversal, (3) diffuse bleeding + documented coagulopathy, or (4) active bleeding with liver disease & a secondary coagulopathy.

Factor VIII preparations: (1) cryoprecipitate is made from single donor and contains fibrinogen, von Willebrand's factor, and factors 8 and 13. (2) factor 8 concentrate is pooled from multiple donors. (3) several recombinant factor 8 products are available.

Factor IX concentrate: Prothrombin complex contains factors II, VII, IX, and X. One unit raises a recipient's activity 1.5%. Factors IX and X are thrombogenic and can cause DIC; therefore, use cautiously in hepatic and vascular disease.

Platelet concentrate: One unit = 5-10 thousand platelets. Platelets are not refrigerated and only survive 7 days. Platelet counts > 50,000/ml are desirable prior to surgery. ABO cross-matching is not necessary. ITP dose 0.1-0.4 U/kg.

Albumin and plasma protein fraction (PPF): 25% salt-poor albumin contains excess sodium (160 mEq Na+/L) and is hyperoncotic compared to plasma. 5% buffered albumin solution is iso-oncotic compared to plasma. PPF contains 88% albumin and 12% globulins and is iso-oncotic compared to plasma.

Testing Blood Prior to Administration

Complete crossmatch - 3 phases (1) Immediate spin phase detects ABO-incompatibility from IgM and takes 5-10 min. (2) Albumin phase takes 15-30 min. (3) Antihuman globulin phase takes 15-30 min. Albumin and antihuman globulin phases detect IgM, IgG, + other antibodies causing hemolytic transfusion reactions.
Unexpected antibody screen uncovers non ABO antibodies (e.g. Kell, Duffy) in recipient's serum. 0.04% of recipients will have a unexpected + antibody screen if no prior transfusion, and 1% will have a positive screen if prior transfusion. This test is important if prior transfusion or pregnancy.
Abbreviated crossmatch: (1) immediate spin alone, or (2) stat crossmatch - omit immediate spin and shorten antihuman globulin and albumin phase to 15 minutes.

Transfusion Reactions

Hemolytic transfusion reactions occur in 1/40,000 transfusions and are usually due to ABO incompatibility. Symptoms: palpitations, abdominal and back pain, syncope, and a sensation of doom. Consider if temperature rises $\geq 2°C$. Immediately stop transfusion, and look for hemoglobinemia and hemoglobinuria. Perform direct antiglobulin (Coomb's test), haptoglobin, peripheral smear, serum bilirubin, and repeat antibody screen + crossmatch. Keep urine output ≥ 100 ml/hour and consider alkalization of urine to limit renal failure. Mannitol is not useful; it increases urine flow by decreasing tubular reabsorption without improving renal perfusion.
Anaphylactic reaction almost exclusively occurs with Anti-IgA antibodies (1/70 people). It usually begins after the first few ml of blood with afebrile flushing, wheezing, cramps, vomiting, diarrhea, and hypotension. Discontinue the transfusion and treat with diphenhydramine, epinephrine and steroids.
Febrile non-hemolytic reactions occur during or soon after initiation of 3-4% of all transfusions, most frequently in multiply transfused or multiparous patients with anti-leukocyte antibodies. Stop transfusion and treat as transfusion reaction.
Urticarial reactions cause local erythema, hives and itching. Further evaluation unnecessary unless fever, chills, or other adverse effects are present. This is the only type of transfusion reaction in which the infusion can continue.
Infections: AIDS, CMV, or hepatitis may be transmitted with blood products.

Blood Products

Component	Indication	Dose	Adverse effects	Special Features
albumin 5%[1]	shock	10-20 ml/kg	rare volume overload, fever, urticaria	stable storage, no filter, no disease transmission
Plasmanate[1]		See above	above and hypotension	above
hetastarch 6% (Hespan)[1]	volume expansion	10-20 ml/kg	prurits, coagulopathy	stable leukopheresis, no disease transmission
Dextran[1]	volume expansion	10 ml/kg	allergy, bleed, renal failure	same as hetastarch
whole blood[2]	hemorrhagic shock	10 ml/kg ↑Hb 1g/dl	transfusion reactions, hemolysis, disease transmission	thrombocytopenia, coagulopathy, leukopenia
packed RBC's[2]	↑O_2 carrying capacity & shock	3 ml/kg ↑Hb 1g/dl	less allergic and febrile reactions than whole blood	same as whole blood; Hct is 70 to 80%, dilute in NS
washed RBC's	↓allergic reactions	3 ml/kg ↑Hb 1g/dl	rare	takes 1 hour to wash and >70% of RBC's lost
leukocyte poor RBC's	99.9% of WBC's are removed	3 ml/kg ↑Hb 1g/dl	rare	use if 2 febrile non-hemolytic reactions to washed RBC's
platelet concentrate	poorly functioning or decreased platelets	1-4 units/ 10 kg	transfusion reactions are rare	no cross-matching, ABO compatibility is preferred
FFP (fresh frozen plasma)	coagulopathy with bleed	10-20 ml/kg	transfusion reactions are rare	no cross-matching, ABO group compatibility preferred

[1]No cross-match needed. [2]For acute hemorrhage, initiate transfusion with 20 ml/kg of whole blood or 10 ml/kg of PRBC's. Request sickle prep neg. blood if sickle cell disease. Avoid mixing blood + D5W or Ringer's lactate due to hemolysis & clotting, respectively.

Hypertension

Hypertensive encephalopathy is the most common presentation of acute hypertension (HTN), with headache, confusion, vomiting, and/or focal neurologic findings. Severe HTN is defined as a systolic BP above the 99th percentile for a given age or >15 mmHg above the 95th percentile. Malignant HTN is severe HTN with retinal changes, papilledema, and widespread fibrinoid necrosis of arterioles.

Age-Based Definition of "Severe" Hypertension:

(Task force on BP in children, Pediatrics 1987; 79:1)

Age	Systolic BP	Diastolic BP
Newborn-7 days	≥ 106	--
1-2 years	≥ 118	≥ 82
3-5 years	≥ 124	≥ 84
6-9 years	≥ 130	≥ 86
10-12 years	≥ 134	≥ 90
13-15 years	≥ 144	≥ 92
16-18 years	≥ 150	≥ 98

Etiology of Pediatric Hypertension (HTN)

- *Renal disease* is the most common cause of both acute and chronic HTN. HTN and encephalopathy (or seizures) may be the initial presentation of acute post-streptococcal glomerulonephritis. Sodium retention and volume expansion occur due to diminished glomerular filtration rate, resulting in an acute rise in BP. Findings in nephritis include hematuria, periorbital edema, & RBC casts.
- *CNS disease*: Cushing's triad of bradycardia, bradypnea, and HTN are found with increased intracranial pressure, and can result from intracerebral tumors, hemorrhage, trauma, or infection.
- *Neuroblastomas* can cause HTN due to increased catecholamine release, similar to neurofibromatosis and pheochromocytoma. This HTN may be episodic, and associated with flushing, palpitations, anxiety, sweating, and chest pain. Cortical adrenal tumors secrete cortisol and can cause HTN.
- *Drug toxicity*: HTN can be due to various mechanisms from steroids, non-steroidal anti-inflammatories, phenylephrine, pseudoephedrine, albuterol, cyclosporine A, and drugs of abuse. Chronic lead toxicity can cause HTN, as can licorice through its mineralocorticoid effects.
- *Aortic coarctation* (CoA) is the most common cause of HTN in the first year of life. CoA also causes up to 2% of secondary HTN in children and adolescents.
- *Other*: Burn victims often exhibit HTN due to sympathetic discharge. 43% of babies with bronchopulmonary dysplasia exhibit HTN.

Drugs in Hypertensive Emergencies

Drug	Dose (max), route, preparation	Mechanism	Onset (Lasts)	Features
captopril (Capoten)	test: 0.01 mg/kg PO, then 0.15 mg/kg PO, double q 2 h until BP control. (max: 4-6 mg/kg/day - bid-tid) Tabs: 12.5, 25, 50, 100 mg	ACE inhibitor	15 min (12h)	useful in renin-induced HTN, side effects include dry cough, rash, angioedema, neutropenia, proteinuria, ↑K+ and creatinine
enalaprilt (Vasotec)	5-10 microg/kg IV q 8-24 hours	ACE inhibitor	1 h (6 h)	see captopril, use test dose - 0.01 mg/kg if no prior use
esmolol (Brevibloc)	500 microg/kg/kg IV over 1st min, then titrate 50-200 microg/kg/min	β-blockade	< 1 min (9min)	can cause or worsen bronchospasm, bradycardia
fenoldopam (Corlopam)	0.1-2.0 microg/kg/min IV infusion	Dopamine-1 agonist	4 min (10 min)	↑ renal flow, & Na+ excretion, contains metabisulfite (allergy)
furosemide (Lasix)	1-4 mg/kg IV	loop diuretic	5 min (3h)	hyperglycemia
labetalol (Normodyne)	Start at 0.2 mg/kg IV; double dose q15 min prn (max: 2-3 mg/kg/dose)	α+ β block in 1:7 ratio	< 1 min (6h)	bronchospasm
nicardipine(Cardene)	0.03mg/kg IV or 1-5 microg/kg/min IV	Ca chn block	2 min (40 min)	↑ICP, ↑HR, ↑V/Q mismatch
nifedipine (Procardia)	0.25-0.50 mg/kg PO/SL (max: 1mg/kg/day) Caps:10,20 mg; Tabs: 30,60,90 mg	Ca channel blocker	2 min (6h)	May ↑ICP, facial flushing, may too rapidly lower pressure causing stroke, or hypoperfusion
nimodipine (Nimotop)	0.35 mg/kg PO (max: 30-60 mg/dose q4-6) Tabs: 30 mg	Ca channel blocker	1 h (9h)	not approved < 12 yr. ↓neuro deficit in subarachnoid bleed
propranolol (Inderal)	0.01-0.1 mg/kg IV over 10min, max 1mg	β-blockade	< 1 min (8h)	bradycardia, bronchospasm
sodium nitroprusside (Nipride)	0.5-8 microg/kg/min IV infusion	arterial & venous dilate	< 1 min (min)	no↓cardiac output, possible cyanide toxicity and ↑ ICP

sec-seconds, min-minutes, h-hours, mo-months, ma-milligrams, µa-micrograms, IV-intravenous, PO-oral, SL-sublingual.

Hypertensive Encephalopathy

BP autoregulation is lost and vasodilation occurs causing cerebral ischemia. Vasodilators in children with HTN and ↑ ICP may be detrimental. Patients with underlying chronic HTN are less likely to develop acute symptoms. Search for underlying disease and end-organ damage in any patient with acute HTN.

Treatment of Hypertensive Encephalopathy (see page 72 for dosing)

- <u>Sodium nitroprusside</u> (*Nipride*) by IV infusion is the drug of choice, due to its rapid onset and short half-life. It is light sensitive. Metabolism produces cyanide which is detoxified to thiocyanate and renally excreted. Nitroprusside also causes cerebral vasodilation and may theoretically increase intracranial pressure. This is the drug of choice for most hypertensive emergencies unless there is a space occupying cranial lesion or significant renal failure.

- <u>Nicardipine</u> is extremely effective for controlled reduction of BP in children and the 2nd most common agent recommended for hypertensive emergencies. It ↓peripheral vascular resistance, has little effect on heart rate and can↑ICP.

- <u>Labetalol</u> (*Normodyne*) is an α + β blocker. It is relatively safe in patients with renal disease and metabolized by the liver. This agent does not ↑ ICP. It is less potent than nicardipine and nitroprusside, produces a reduction in cardiac output, and may cause bronchospasm and worsen congestive heart failure.

- <u>Nifedipine</u> **Use cautiously** as this drug can have uncontrolled BP lowering effects producing cerebral or coronary ischemia.

- <u>Fenoldopam</u> (*Corlopam*) dopamine 1 receptor agonist. Titratable IV with good safety profile

---

Immunizations

CHILD IMMUNIZATION SCHEDULE*					Months						Years	
Age	Birth	1	2	4	6	12	15	18	24	4-6	11-12	14-16
Hepatitis B	HB1	← only if mother HbsAg(-)										
		HB-2			HB-3							
DPT†			DTP	DTP	DTP		DTP			DTP	Td	
H influenza b			Hib	Hib	Hib	Hib						
S.pneumonia			PCV	PCV	PCV	PCV						
Polio§			IPV	IPV		IPV				IPV		
MMR						MMR				MMR		
Varicella						Varicella						
Hepatitis A¶										HA (some areas)		

*2002 schedule from the CDC, ACIP, AAP, & AAFP, see CDC website (www.cdc.gov). Annual influenza vaccine recommended for children >6 months old with risk factors such as asthma, cardiac disease, sickle cell diseases, HIV, diabetes. †Acellular form preferred for all DTP doses. §Inactivated form (IPV) preferred for all doses in the US. ¶Recommended for selected high-risk areas, consult local public health authorities.

Hepatitis B Exposure

Type of exposure	Status of source is	Treatment if exposed patient is	
		Unvaccinated	Vaccinated
percutaneous or mucosal	HBsAg +	HBIG, HBV	HBV & HBIG if exposed HBsAb -
known source	high risk for HBsAg +	HBV and HBIG if source HBsAg +	HBV & HBIG if source HBsAg+ & exposed HBsAb-
known source	low risk for HBsAg +	HBV	none
unknown	unknown	HBV	none
sex / perinatal	HBsAg +	HBIG, HBV	none
house/work	HBsAg +	none	none

HBIG = hepatitis B immune globulin. Dose 0.06 ml/kg IM
HBV = hepatitis B vaccine. Dose: 0.5 ml IM in deltoid initially, repeat in 1 & 6 mo.
Hepatitis C exposure: Administer immune serum globulin (ISG) 0.06 ml/kg IM.
Hepatitis A exposure: Administer ISG 0.02 ml/kg IM for exposure through close personal contact, employee at day care center, or contaminated food within 2 wks.

Tetanus Immunization

Prior immunization	Tetanus prone wound	Non tetanus prone wound
Uncertain or <3	DT[1], TIG[2]	dT[1]
3 or more	dT if >5y since last dose	dT if >10y since last dose

[1]dT if ≥7 y and DT if <7 y (D contains 2X the diphtheria dose of d). [2]Tetanus immune globulin
Dose of tetanus globulin (TIG): Age ≥ 7 y: 250 units IM at site other than for dT.
Age <7 y: 4 units/kg, although 250 units IM may be appropriate since the same amount of toxin will be produced in the child's body regardless of size.

Postexposure Rabies Prophylaxis (*Ann Emerg Med* 1999; 33: 590.)
Rabies prophylaxis only indicated if bite or other salivary exposure from bat or carnivore. No prophylaxis is needed if nonsalivary or if bird, reptile, or rodent. If questions arise regarding prophylaxis and local and state health department unavailable call CDC at **404-639-1050** (days), **404-639-2888** (nights & weekends)

- (1) Human diploid cell vaccine (HDCV) **Or** (2) Rabies vaccine adsorbed (RVA) **Or** (3) Purified chick embryo cell vaccine (PCEC) dose - 1 ml IM, on days 0, 3, 7, 14, & 28. Administer vaccine in deltoid, not buttock. **PLUS**
- RIG (rabies immune globulin) dose - 20 IU/kg with full dose infiltrated SC around the wound (if possible) and remainder IM distal to the site of RIG. Do not give near the site of the 1st HDCV injection.

Is animal a dog or cat?

		YES	NO, other
Was animal captured?	NO, escaped	Give RIG & HDCV only if rabies risk for given species in locale.	Treat with RIG and full course of HDCV.
	YES, captured	Observe animal for 10 days. If abnormal behavior, sacrifice and treat patient with RIG & vaccine. Discontinue treatment if animal pathology negative for rabies.	Sacrifice animal and begin RIG and vaccine. Discontinue treatment if pathology negative for rabies.

Adult Health Care Worker Exposure to Human Immunodeficiency Virus (HIV)

- Highest risk for transmission of HIV: (1) scalpel or needle visibly contaminated with patient's blood, (2) needle placed directly in vein or artery, (3) deep puncture or wound to health care worker (4) terminal illness in source patient.
- ZDV reduces transmission by ~ 79%. Begin prophylaxis ≤ 2-8 h from exposure.

Provisional Public Health Service Recommendations for Chemoprophylaxis after Occupational Exposure to HIV.

Exposure	Source Material	Prophylaxis?	Drug Regimen [1]
Percutaneous	Blood -Highest risk[2]	Recommend	ZDV + 3TC + IDV
HIV risk	Increased risk[2]	Recommend	ZDV + 3TC ± IDV
~ 0.3%	No increased risk[2]	Offer	ZDV + 3TC
	Fluid has visible blood or		
	other infectious fluid[3]	Offer	ZDV + 3TC
	Other fluid (e.g. urine)	Do not offer	
Mucous	Blood	Offer	ZDV + 3TC ± IDV
membrane	Fluid has visible blood or		
HIV risk	other infectious fluid[3]	Offer	ZDV + 3TC
~ 0.1%	Other fluid (e.g. urine)	Do not offer	
Skin with ↑	Blood	Offer	ZDV + 3TC ± IDV
risk[4]	Fluid has visible blood or		
HIV risk	other infectious fluid	Offer	ZDV ± 3TC
< 0.1%	Other fluid (e.g. urine)	Do not offer	

1 ZDV – zidovudine, 3TC – lamivudine, IDV - indinavir
2 Highest risk – ↑blood volume (e.g. deep injury with ↑diameter hollow needle) AND
  blood with ↑ titer HIV (e.g. source patient is end-stage, or has↑viral load)
  Increased risk - Exposure to ↑blood volume or blood with ↑HIV titer
  No increased risk - Neither exposure to large blood volume or high HIV titer
3 Semen, vaginal secretions, CSF, synovial, pleural, peritoneal, pericardial, amniotic fluid
4 Increased risk (for skin) = exposures with high HIV titer, prolonged contact, extensive
  area, or area in which skin integrity is visibly compromised.
  JAMA 1999; 281: 931; CDC. *MMWR.* 1996; 45: 468)

Protocol and Drug Dosing for HIV Exposure

♦ Draw HIV, CBC, liver+renal function, βhCG ± hepatitis exposure work up (pg 74)
♦ Repeat CBC, liver + renal tests at 2 weeks, and HIV at 6 and 12 weeks, + 12 mo.

zidovudine(ZDV)	200 mg PO tid Or 300 mg BID X 4 weeks[1]
lamivudine(3TC)	150 mg PO bid X 4 weeks[1]
indinavir (IDV)	800 mg PO tid X 4 weeks (may substitute snelfinivir 750 mg PO tid)

Most common short term side effects: *ZDV* - GI, fatigue, headache; *3TC* - GI, pancreatitis, *IDV* - GI, high bilirubin, and kidney stones (may be limited by drinking ≥ 1.5 L H2O/day).
1 If ZDV plus 3TC regimen may substitute *Combivir* (1 tab PO BID).
  JAMA 1999; 281: 931; CDC. *MMWR.* 1996; 45: 468

Child & Adolescent Non-Occupational HIV Post-exposure Prophylaxis (PEP)

Prerequisites

(1) offer PEP only if patient not HIV + (2) do not give if source HIV neg. or insignificant exposure [kiss] (3) must be voluntary & require patient & caretaker to compete 28 d regiment/follow-up (4) Notify all that PEP is not cure & efficacy is unknown (6) if risky sex/IV drugs, patient agrees to therapy and follow up to ↓ risk.

Suggested Regimens & Goal

- Provide 1st dose within 1 h of presentation, 72 h of exposure. Treat X 28 days.
- Provide ≥ 72 hour med supply & refer to appropriate follow up within 72h ED visit
- <u>HIV source med regimen unknown</u>: AZT + lamivudine + (indinavir or nelfinavir)
- <u>HIV source regimen known</u>: NRTI + protease inhibitor different from source's regimen. Do not combine (1) *d4T* with *AZT* or *ddC* OR (2) *ddl* with *ddC*
- **High HIV risk & unknown HIV status:** *Significant exposure*: AZT + Epivir, + indinavir or nelfinavir. *Unclear significance*: AZT + Epivir ± add protease inhibitor.
- **Low HIV risk/unknown HIV status:** *Significant exposure*, AZT + Epivir, + indinavir or nelfinavir. *Unclear significance, <u>consider</u>* AZT + Epivir ± add protease inhibitor.

<u>High risk HIV source</u> – IV, bloody needle or sharp from area ↑ HIV seroprevalence, IV drug use sharps, male-male sex, multiple partners, sex with HIV+ person, sex assault from unknown HIV status assailant, sex for drugs or money. <u>Significant exposure</u> – unprotected anal/vaginal intercourse, IV drugs use, exposure to semen or blood on mucosal or nonintact surfaces <u>Unclear significance exposure</u> – oral sex, semen or blood on healing wound, bites, sharing personal hygiene equipment.

Pediatric HIV PEP Doses for Antiretrovirals[1]

Nucleoside Reverse Transcriptase Inhibitors (NRTI) (1st line-*AZT, Epivir, Combivir*)	
Abacavir *Ziagen*	3mo-16y: 8 mg/kg up to 300 mg PO bid, >16y: 300mg PO bid
Combivir *AZT/Epivir*	Only available > 16 years at 150 mg PO bid
Didanosine *ddl/Videx*	90-150 mg/m² PO bid: adolescent< 60 kg: 125 mg PO bid, > 60 kg: 200 mg PO bid
Lamivudine *Epivir*	3mo-16y: 4 mg/kg PO bid; > 16y: 150 mg PO bid
Stavudine d4T/*Zerit*	< 30kg: 1mg/kg bid; 30-60kg: 30 mg bid; >60kg 40 mg PObid
Zalcitabine *Hivid/ddC*	0.005-0.01 mg/kg PO q 8h; adolescents: 0.75 mg PO tid
Zidovudine *AZT/ZDV*	3mo-12y: 160 mg/m² PO q6h; > 12y: 300 mg PO bid
Protease Inhibitors (1st line-*Crixivan, Viracept*)	
Amprenavir *Agenerae*	4-12y or 13-16y + < 50 kg: 22.5 mg/kg PO bid or 17 mg/kg PO tid; 13-16 + > 50 kg OR > 16y: 1.4 g PO bid
Indinavir *Crixivan*	Only recommended > 16 y: 800 mg PO q 8h
Lopinavir/ritonavir *Kaletra*	6mo-12y: 7-15 kg: 12 mg/kg bid; 15-40 kg: 10 mg/kg bid > 40 kg OR > 12 y: 5 ml or 3 capsules PO bid
Nelfinavir *Viracept*	2-13y: 20-30 mg/kg bid; > 13y: 750 mg PO tid or 1.25g bid
Saquinavir *Fortovase*	Only recommended > 16 y: 1.2 g PO tid after meals
Nucleoside reverse Transcriptase Inhibitor & Protease Inhibitor Combination	
Trizivir	(ZDV + lamivudine + abacavir) > 13y > 40 kg: 1 PO bid

[1] max dose is equivalent to highest dose for oldest age   *Pediatrics* 2001; 108: e38.

Empiric Antimicrobial Therapy

Acne vulgaris *Retin A and Differin not approved < 12 years old*	• <u>No or mild inflammation</u> – tretinoin (*Retin A*) 0.025-0.1% cream. **OR** adapalene (*Differin*) 0.1% cream or gel Apply qhs • <u>Moderate-severe</u> – (*Erygel/Eryderm* 2-3% **or** *Clindagel* applied bid) **AND** benzoyl peroxide (BP) gel/cream qd-bid ± **ADD** (*Cleocin* **OR** doxycycline PO).Use only ≥ 12 y & ≥ 45 kg *BenzaClin* or *Benzamycin* (BP + clindamycin or erythromycin)
Anthrax exposure	See page 17 for exposure prophylaxis and disease treatment
Appendicitis *regimens are for suspected perforation (e.g. pain > 36-48 hours, temp > 101, diffusely tender)*	• (ampicillin 100-200 mg/kg/d IV divided q 6h [max 12 g/d] **and** gentamicin 7.5 mg/kg/d IV [q 8h] **and** clindamycin 25-40 mg/kg/d IV divided q 8h [max dose q 8h [max 4.8 g/d]) • **OR** *Unasyn* 100-200 mg/kg/d IV divided q6h (max dose – ampicillin 12 g/d) **OR** *Timentin* 200-300 mg/kg/d of ticarcillin IV (4-6h) [max dose 18 g/d] **OR** cefoxitin 100-160 mg/kg/d IV (q 4-6h) [max 12g/d]. Continue all regimens until afebrile X 48-72 hours or total of 10-14 days if severe infection.
Ascaris lumbricoides roundworm	• mebendazole (*Vermox*) 100 mg PO bid X 3d **OR** albendazole 400 mg PO > 13 kg, 200 mg ≤ 13 kg **OR** pyrantel pamoate (*PinX*) 11 mg/kg X 1 (max 1g). Cap-180 mg; Susp:50 mg/5 ml
Bite cat/dog/rat	• <u>All bites 1st agent</u> - *Augmentin* 45 mg/kg/d PO (bid) X 10 days • <u>cat</u> – cefuroxime 30 mg/kg/d PO **OR** if > 8 y may use doxycycline 4 mg/kg/d divided bid (max 200 mg/d) X 10 days • <u>dog</u> – clindamycin + *Septra* PO (see dose pg 84,85) X 10 d • <u>rat</u> – if > 8 years: doxycycline 4 mg/kg/d PO (bid) X 10 days • <u>snake</u> – ceftriaxone 50 mg/kg IV/IM qd (max dose 2 g/d) • <u>Infected/Inpatient</u> – *Unasyn* 100-200 mg/kg/d IV divide q6h IV (max – ampicillin 12 g/d) **OR** IV regimen of above choices
Bite – human	• <u>Outpatient</u> - *Augmentin* 45 mg/kg/d PO (bid) X 10 days • <u>Inpatient</u> – *Unasyn* 100-200 mg/kg/d IV (q 6h) [max 12g/d] **OR** cefoxitin 100-160 mg/kg/d IV (q 4-6h) [max 12g/d] **OR** (*Cleocin* 25-40 mg/kg/d IV (q 6-8h) [max 4.8 g/d] **and** *Septra* 15-20 mg/kg/d IV or PO (q6-8h) of TMP [max TMP 320mg/d])
Bordatella pertussis	• erythromycin 40 mg/kg/d PO (qid)X 14 d (max 2 g/d) Only ↓ disease if give in catarrhal stage. Can ↓ recurrence + transmission. If give < 6 weeks old, pyloric stenosis risk.
Bronchitis	See CDC/AAP recommendations page 91.
Campylobacter	• diarrhea - erythromycin 40mg/kg/d PO (qid) X 5d max 2g
Candida	• <u>Thrush (neonate)</u> – nystatin 1 ml/cheek qid: susp:100,000 U/ml. (Child) 500,000U PO qid until clear 48h. 500,000U/tab • <u>Oral</u> – *Diflucan* 6 mg/kg X1, + 3 mg/kg X 14 d (21 days for esophageal), (if < 14 day old, give dose q72 h - not q d)
Cat scratch disease	azithromycin 10 mg/kg PO (max 500) + 5 mg/kg X4d (max 250mg) **OR** *Septra* 12mg/kg/d TMP PO (bid) [max TMP 320mg/d]

Cellulitis bite	See specific animal or human bite above
Cellulitis face	• If mild, immunized, no sinusitis,& well-appearing – dicloxacillin **OR** Augmentin **OR** 1st gen cephalosporin PO (page 84) • Ill or unimmunized or sinusitis - cefotaxime (*Claforan*) 100-200 mg/kg/d IV (q 6-8h) [max 12g/d] **OR** cefuroxime (*Zinacef*) 75-150 mg/kg/d IV (q 8h) [max 9g/day]
Cellulitis trunk or extremity	• Mild – cephalexin **OR** dicloxacillin **OR** erythromycin **OR** clarithromycin X 7-10 d **OR** azithromycin PO X 5 d (dose pg 84) • Mod-Severe - oxacillin **OR** nafcillin 100-200 mg/kg/d IV (q 6h) [max 12 g/d] **OR** cephazolin 100 mg/kg/d (q6-8h) [max 6 g/d]
Chlamydia > 12y *urethritis, cervicitis*	• azithromycin 1 g PO **OR** doxycycline 100 mg PO bid x 7-10 d **OR** erythromycin 500 mg PO qid x 7-10d **+** treat gonorrhea
C. difficile	Clostridium difficile - See pseudomembranous colitis
Conjunctivitis	• Neonate – if gonorrhea - cefotaxime 100 mg/kg/d IV (bid) X 1-2 d **ADD** erythromycin PO (page 84) for Chlamydia • > 2 weeks – ciprofloxacin (*Ciloxan*) 0.3% sol'n 1-2 drops q2h X 2d, then q4h X 5d **OR** erythromycin (*Ilotycin*) 0.5% oint apply q 4h until clear X 2d **OR** gentamicin (*Garamycin*) 0.3% oint/sol'n apply q 3-4h X 7-10d, **OR** *Polytrim* sol'n 1 drop q 3h X 7-10 d **OR** tobramycin (*Tobrex*) 0.3% sol'n/oint [gent dose]
Cutaneous larval migrans	• albendazole (*Albenza*) 15 mg/kg mo PO X 1 (max 400) [200 mg tab] **OR** ivermectin (*Stromectol*) 200 microg/kg PO X 1 **OR** thiabendazole (*Mintezol*) 50 mg/kg/d (bid) PO (max 3 g/d)
Diarrhea	See Salmonella, Shigella, E. coli, Campylobacter, Yersinia, Traveler
E. coli diarrhea	• Septra 8 mg/kg/d of TMP PO (bid) [max dose 320 mgTMP/d] **OR** cefixime 8 mg/kg/d PO (qd) [max 400 mg/d] X 5 d. STEC Shiga toxin E. coli (0157:H7) does not improve with antibiotics
Ehrlichiosis	See doxycycline dose for Rky Mt. Spotted Fever OR Rifampin
Endocarditis	• Unknown organism - (Penicillin G 150,000 U/kg/d divide q 4-6h [max 24 million U/d] **or** ampicillin 200 mg/kg/d (q 4h) [max 12 g/d] **AND** nafcillin or oxacillin 100-200 mg/kg/d (q 6h) [max 12 g/d] **AND** gentamicin 6-7.5 mg/kg/d divided q 8h) IV X 4-6 weeks. Alter regimen once specific organism known • Penicillin allergic – gentamicin 6-7.5 mg/kg/d divided q 8h **AND** vancomycin 30 mg/kg/d divided q 12 h (max 2 g/d)
Entamoeba histolytica	• metronidazole (*Flagyl*) 35-50 mg/kg/d PO/IV (q 8h) X 10d • followed by iodoquinol 40 mg/kg/d (tid after meal) [max 2g/d] X 20 d **OR** paromomycin 30 mg/kg/d (tid) X 10 d [max 1.5g/d]
Enterobius vermicularis pinworms	• mebendazole (*Vermox*) 100 mg PO X 1, repeat in 2 wks **OR** albendazole (*Albenza*) 15 mg/kg PO X 1 (max 400), **OR** pyrantel pamoate(*PinX*) 11mg/kg X1(max 1g):Cap-62.5;50/5ml
Giardia lamblia	• furazolidone (*Furoxon*) 8 mg/kg/d divided qid PO X 10 d (max 400 mg/day) **OR** metronidazole (*Flagyl*) 15 mg/kg/d (tid) X 5d **OR** albendazole (*Albenza*) (> 6y) 400 mg PO qd X 5d

Gonorrhea – > 12 years old	• Uncomplicated disease (cervicitis/urethritis, not PID, arthritis, epididymitis) cefixime 400 mg PO, **OR** ceftriaxone 125 mg IM **OR** azithromycin 2 g PO (also treat *Chlamydia*)
Herpes simplex	• <u>mucocutaneous – (including gingivostomatitis)</u> acyclovir 75-80 mg/kg/d (5X/day) X 7-10 d (max 1.2 g/d); • <u>encephalitis</u> – acyclovir 30 mg/kg/d over 1 hour IV (tid) X 21 d
Herpes zoster	• See *varicella* for chicken pox disease/exposure manage • <u>disseminated or immunocompromised or severe chicken pox</u> - acyclovir 30 mg/kg/d over 1-2 hours IV (tid) X 7 d
Hookworm	• mebendazole (*Vermox*) 100 mg PO bid X 3 days or 500 mg PO X 1, **OR** albendazole (*Albenza*) 15 mg/kg PO X 1 (max 400 mg) pyrantel pamoate 11 mg/kg/d X 3 d (max 1 g/d)
Impetigo	• mupirocin (*Bactroban*) apply tid **OR** cefadroxil **OR** cephalexin **OR** dicloxacillin **OR** erythromycin X 7 days (dose page 84)
Influenza treatment *start within* *48h of* *symptoms*	• <u>Influenza A</u> – amantadine (> 1y) **OR** rimantidine (> 14 y) (*Flumadine*) 5 mg/kg/d (bid) X 7d (max 150 mg/d):Tab 100mg, Susp 50 mg/5ml • <u>Influenza A or B</u> – oseltamivir (*Tamiflu*) (> 1 y) - ≤ 15 kg: 30 mg PO bid [max 60 mg/d]; > 15-23 kg: 45 mg PO bid; > 23-40 kg: 60 mg PO bid; > 40 kg: 75 mg PO bid X 5 days. **OR** zanamivir (*Relenza*) (only approved ≥ 7 years) 2 inhalations (one 5 mg blister/inhalation) given bid X 5 days. Use bronchodilator before using *Relenza* if bronchospasm.
Influenza prophylaxis	• <u>Influenza A</u> - amantadine or rimantidine – use same dose as treatment qd (may use rimantidine > 1 y for prophylaxis) Continue for 2-6 weeks – variable recommendations. • <u>Influenza A or B</u> - oseltamivir (*Tamiflu*) only approved for prophylaxis > 13 years old: 75 mg PO qd X 7 days to 6 week.
IV catheter line infection	• vancomycin 60 mg/kg/d IV [q6h] **AND** gentamicin 7.5 mg/kg/d IV [q 8h] **ADD** *Fortaz* 150 mg/kg/d IV (q 8h) if neutropenic
Lice	See *pediculus humanus capitis* (pediculosis)
Lyme Disease *See page 89 for* *detail regarding* *early vs late* *disease*	• <u>Early</u> (all PO) – doxycycline 4 mg/kg/d (bid) [max 200mg/d] if > 8y amoxicillin 50 mg/kg/d (tid) **OR** cefuroxime 30 mg/ kg/d (bid) X 21 d (30 d arthritis, Bell's palsy,multiple ECM) • <u>Early disease with meningitis or carditis or more than mild early arthritis or Late disease</u> – ceftriaxone 75-100 mg/kg/d IV/IM (max 2 g) **OR** penicillin G 200,000 to 400,000 U/kg/d IV (max 24 million U/d) divided q 4h X 14-28 days.
Mastoiditis	• <u>Acute</u> - cefuroxime 150 mg/kg/d IV/IM (q8h) **OR** ceftriaxone 50 mg/kg/d IV/IM (qd) X 10 days • <u>Chronic</u> – *Timentin* 200-300 mg/kg/d (q 4-6h) **OR** ceftazidime 100-150 mg/kg/d IV/IM (q 8h) **OR** cefepime (*Maxipime*) 100-150 mg/kg/d (q 8-12h) IV **PLUS** surgery may be required.

Measles	• <u>Exposure</u> - Prophylax if *susceptible* & > 12 mo old & exposed. *Susceptible* = all persons unless had documented measles, born < 1957, lab evidence immunity, or completed appropriate live-virus vaccination. **DO NOT** give if neomycin allergy, TB, immunosuppressed, steroids, heme cancer, pregnant, ≤ 3 mo from blood/Immunoglobulin use. • <u>Use</u> of live vaccine ≤ 72 h after exposure prevents disease. Use monovalent vaccine if 6-12 mo old. Use *Immune globulin* (IG) if immunosuppressed or pregnant:(1) 0.25 ml/kg (max 15 ml) IM within 6 d exposure.(2) Double (max 15 ml) if immunocompromised. (3) Give measles vaccine ≥ 5 mo after IG.
Meningitis	• <u>0-2 months</u> – (ampicillin 100-200 (300 if Gp B strep) mg/kg/d IV (q 8-12h) **AND** [gentamicin 5-7.5 mg/kg/d (q8-12) or cefotaxime 100-200 mg/kg/d (q 6-12)] • <u>> 2 months</u> – (cefotaxime 200-300 mg/kg/d (q 6h) [max 12 g/d] use higher 300 mg/kg/d if pneumococcal meningitis **or** ceftriaxone 100 mg/kg/d IV (qd) [max 4 g/d]) **AND** vancomycin 60 mg/kg/d (q 6h) [max 1 g/dose]
Meningococcemia	See *Neisseria meningitidis* disease
Neisseria meningitidis	• <u>Exposure</u> –Rifampin 10 mg/kg PO q12h X 4 (Max dose 600 mg) **OR** ceftriaxone 125-250 mg IM **OR** May substitute sulfisoxazole if organism sulfa sensitive **OR** ciprofloxacin 500 mg X 1 in adults. Treat household, day care, or nursery contacts within 24h of case, older children/adults if kissed, shared food or drink. Medical person exposed to secretions. • <u>Disease</u> – Penicillin G 250,000 U/kg/d divide q 4h IV X 7days.
Neutropenic fever	See Infectious Disease Society America guidelines page 67.
Omphalitis	• <u>≤ 2 months</u> – oxacillin or nafcillin 150 mg/kg/d (divide qid) **AND** gentamicin 7.5 mg/kg/d [q 8h] • <u>> 2 months</u> – cefotaxime 200 mg/kg/d (divide q 6h) **OR** Unasyn 200 mg/kg/d (divide q 6h)
Onychomycosis	See tinea unguium
Osteomyelitis	• nafcillin **OR** oxacillin 100-150 mg/kg/d IV (q 4-6h) **OR** vancomycin 40 mg/kg/d IV [q 8h] **OR** if > 2 months clindamycin 25-40 mg/kg/d IV (q 8h) [max 4.8 g/d] • **ADD** cefotaxime 100-200 mg/kg/d (q 6-8h) if ≤ 2 months or if gram negative bacteria on gram stain.
Otitis externa	• *Cortisporin otic* 3 gtts qid **OR** *Cipro HC otic* (> 1 y) 3 gtt bid **OR** *Floxin otic* (> 1 y) 5 gtt bid **OR** *Otobiotic* 4 gtts qid **OR** *Pediotic* 3-4 gtts qid **OR** *Vosol HC* (> 3 y) 3-4 gtts qid: 7-10 d • <u>Mod-severe</u> – dicloxacillin **OR** *Keflex* **OR** *Augmentin* page 84 • If chronic, ill or pseudomonas suspected – see chronic mastoiditis antibiotic choices and doses.
Otitis Media	See CDC working group recommendations page 90.

Pediculus humanus capitis (pediculosis or lice)	• permethrin 1% (*Nix*) applied to hair/scalp X 10 min, may repeat in 1-2 weeks **OR** permethrin 5% cream (*Elimite*) applied overnight **OR** lindane (*Kwell, Scabene*) 1% shampoo applied for 4 minutes, then rinse **OR** lindane 1% lotion apply overnight > 8 h, repeat in 1 week [avoid if < 2 y or seizures] • <u>resistance or treatment failure:</u> *Septra* PO X 3 d, repeat in 1 week, most effective if combined with permethrin **OR** ivermectin (*Stromectol*) 200 microg/kg PO or as an 0.8% solution [ivermectin not approved < 15 kg] **OR** malathion (*Ovide*) 0.5% shampoo X 10 min, reapply in 1 week.
Pelvic Inflam-matory disease *Age > 12 years*	• <u>outpatient</u> – ceftriaxone 250 mg IM X 1 **AND** doxycycline 100 mg PO bid X 14 d. • <u>inpatient</u> – (I) ([cefoxitin 2g IV q 6h or cefotetan 2 g IV q 12h] **plus** doxycycline 100 mg PO/IV q 12 h) **OR** (II) (gentamicin 2.5 mg/kg IV q 8h **and** clindamycin 900 mg IV q 8 h). Continue until well X 48 h then doxycycline 100 mg PO bid X 14 d ± **ADD** *Cleocin* or *Flagyl* PO (dose page 84,85) if abscess, recurrence or post op.
Perforation bowel	• See appendicitis perforation regimens **OR** meropenem (*Merrem*) if > 3 months: 60 mg/kg/d IV (q 8h) [max 6 g/d]
Peritonsillar	abscess – see retropharyngeal abscess
Pinworm	See *Enterobius vermicularis*
Pharyngitis *Gp A strep.*	• benzathine penicillin 25,000 U/kg IM (max 1.2 mill U) X 1 **OR** penicillin **OR** 1st gen cephalosporin **OR** clindamycin X 10 d. (see PO dose page 84). Not erythromycin - 48% resistance.
Pneumonia *aspiration*	• (clindamycin 25-40 mg/kg/d IV divided q 8h [max dose 4.8 g/d] or *Timentin* 200-300 mg/kg/d of ticarcillin IV (4-6h) [max dose 18 g/d]) **AND** gentamicin 7.5 mg/kg/d [q 8h])
Pneumonia	• 0-4 weeks – ampicillin 100-200 mg/kg/d IV (q 8-12h) **AND** [gentamicin 2.5 mg/kg/dose (q 12-18 h if < 7 days or < 1.2 kg or q 8 h if > 7 days + > 2 kg) **or** cefotaxime 50 mg/kg/dose]. If Chlamydia, add erythromycin page 84. • > 4 weeks – 3 months – ampicillin 100-200 mg/kg/d (q 6h) **AND** cefotaxime 200 mg/kg/d (q 6h) [max 12 g/d]. If *B. pertussis* or Chlamydia add erythromycin page 84. • > 3 months – (A) inpatient– (cefuroxime 100-150 mg/kg/d (q 8h) **or** cefotaxime 100-200 mg/kg/d (q 6-8h) [max 12 g/d] **or** ceftriaxone 50 mg/kg/d (qd) [max 2 g/d]) **AND** (azithromycin or clarithromycin **or** erythromycin) see dose page 84. • > 3 months – (B) outpatient– azithromycin **OR** clarithromycin **OR** erythromycin (esp. > 5-7 y) **OR** *Augmentin* if Mycoplasma not suspected X 10 days– see dose pg 84 (azithromycin 5 d)
Pseudomem-braneous colitis	• metronidazole (*Flagyl*) 30 mg/kg/d PO (q 6h) [max 4 g/d] **OR** vancomycin 40 mg/kg/d PO (q 6h) [max 2 g/d] X 7-10 days

Pyelonephritis	See urinary tract infection
Q fever	• See page 18.
Retropharyngeal abscess	Same regimen for retropharyngeal, lateral (para) pharyngeal, submandibular/sublingual (Ludwig's), peritonsillar abscesses • clindamycin 25-40 mg/kg/d (q 8h) [max 4.8 g/d] **OR** _Unasyn_ 200 mg/kg/d (q 6h) [max 8 g/d] **OR** cefoxitin 100-160 mg/kg/d IV (q 4-6h) [max 12g/d]. Surgery usually required.
Rocky Mountain Spotted Fever	• doxycycline 4.4 mg/kg/d PO or IV (bid) [max 200 mg/d] **OR** chloramphenical 50-75 mg/kg/d IV (q6h) [max 4 g/d] until afebrile X 3 d or 7-10 d. If ≤ 8 y, consider risks of doxycycline (teeth stain) vs. chloramphenical (bone marrow suppression).
Roundworm	See _Ascaris lumbricoides_
Salmonella	• Sepsis or focal infection – cefotaxime 100-200 (225-300 if meningitis) mg/kg/d IV (q 6-8h) X 7-10 days. • Diarrhea – treat only if septic, age < 3 months, immuno-compromised, or bacteremia. _Septra_ – 10 mg/kg/d of TMP (bid) X 14 days. (see page 85)
Scabies	• permethrin 5% cream (_Elimite_) to entire body (+ scalp in infants) overnight then wash off **OR** lindane (_Kwell, Scabene_) 1% lotion to body overnight then wash off [avoid if < 2 y or seizures] **OR** crotamiton (_Eurax_) apply chin to feet, repeat in 24 h, wash off in 48 h **OR** ivermectin (_Stromectol_) 200 µg/kg PO [ivermectin not approved < 15 kg] **OR** 6% sulfur in petroleum cream applied overnight
Sepsis	Treat per meningitis or neutropenia depending on source
Septic arthritis	• **(nafcillin or oxacillin 100-150 mg/kg/d IV [q 4-6h])** • **AND (cefotaxime 100-200 mg/kg/d [q 6-8h] or gentamicin 7.5 mg/kg/d [q 8h]). Substitute** vancomycin 40 mg/kg/d IV [q 8h] for nafcillin/oxacillin if methicillin resistance possible.
Shigella diarrhea	• _Septra_ 8 mg/kg/d of TMP PO (bid) [max dose 320 mgTMP/d] **OR** cefixime 8 mg/kg/d PO (qd) [max 400 mg/d] X 5 days
Sinusitis _See page 91 for AAP/CDC recommendation regarding diagnosis and treatment_	CDC recommendations _Pediatrics_ 2001; 108: 798. • amoxicillin 45 mg/kg/d **OR** amoxicillin/_Augmentin_ 90 mg/kg/d **OR** cefdinir 14 mg/kg/d (qd-bid), **OR** cefuroxime 30 mg/kg/d (bid) **OR** cefpodoxime 10 mg/kg/d (qd) See doses page 84. • If allergy to above, clarithromycin **OR** azithromycin **OR** clindamycin (dose page 84). Continue for 10-28 days (azithromycin 5 days) or until symptom free, then 7 days. • If periorbital/orbital cellulitis ceftriaxone IV 100 mg/kg/d (bid) **OR** _Unasyn_ 200 mg/kg/d (q6h) **ADD** vancomycin 60 mg/kg/d IV (qid) if drug resistant _S. pneumoniae_ +CT & ENT consult
Submandibular	abscess – see retropharyngeal abscess
Tick bite	• doxycycline 3 mg/kg (max 200 mg) PO single dose if Lyme endemic area & > 8 yo. Consider risks/benefits ≤ 8 yo.

Tinea capitis or kerion – *oral steroids may↓ kerion scarring*	• griseofulvin 10-20 mg/kg/d PO (bid) (microsize) **OR** 5-10 mg/kg/d PO (bid-qd) ultramicrosize X 4-6wks **OR** itraconazole (*Sporanox*) 3-5 mg/kg/d X 4-5 wks **OR** fluconazole (*Diflucan*) 6 mg/kg/d PO X 3-6 wks **OR** terbinafine (*Lamisil*) PO qd X 4-6 weeks (see dose page 85) *Sporanox/Diflucan/Lamisil* not FDA approved, recommended if fail griseofulvin. *Derm Clin* 1998; 527
Tinea corporis, cruris, pedis	• Topical options - butenafine apply bid-qd, ciclopirox bid, clotrimazole bid, econazole bid, haloprogin, ketoconazole qd, miconazole bid, naftifine qd, oxiconazole qd-bid, terbinafine
Tinea unguium *Only griseofulvin FDA approved Monitor others closely*	• griseofulvin 10-20 mg/kg/d PO (micro) **OR** 5-10 mg/kg/d PO (bid-qd) ultramicrosize X 3-6 mo **OR** itraconazole (*Sporanox*) 5 mg/kg/d X 1 week q month X3(fingers) & 1 week q month X 4 months (toes) **OR** terbinafine PO qd X 6 weeks (finger), X 12 weeks (toes) – see page 85 for dose.
Tinea versicolor	• topical selenium sulfide,clotrimazole,econazole, **OR** hal progin • oral - itraconazole 3-5 mg/kg/d X 15 d PO if extensive lesions
Traveler diarrhea	See E. coli antibiotic regimens
Tularemia	See page 79 for prophylaxis and treatment.
Urinary tract infection	See page 92 for expert guidelines regarding management including antibiotic choices.
Varicella disease	• Acyclovir (*Zovirax*) 20 mg/kg PO qid X 5d (max dose 800 mg) Use if > 12 y, or chronic cutaneous/pulmonary disorder, or on chronic salicylates or on steroids ± 2ⁿᵈ household case. Pregnancy is not indication. (effective within 48 h of exposure) • See page 79 for management of zoster or varicella in immunocompromised host.
Varicella exposure	• Varicella immune globulin (VZIG) if same household, playmate, hospital exposure, newborn below exposure to immunocompromised (also HIV+) no prior chicken pox, susceptible pregnant women, newborn with mom's chicken pox onset ≤ 5 days pre to 2 days post delivery, or hospitalized premature infants ≥ 28 weeks whose mom has no prior chicken pox, is seronegative or newborn < 28 weeks regardless of mom's history exposed to varicella. Give VZIG within 96 h exposure. • VZIG dose *Newborn*: 125U IM *Older*: 125U/10 kg (max 625 U) • Vaccine – administer vaccine 0.5 ml IM to all exposed susceptible children within 72 hours (± up to 120 hours) • Acyclovir – administer 7 day course if VZIG contraindicated.
Ventricular CSF shunt infection	• (vancomycin 60 mg/kg/d IV [q6h] or nafcillin 150-200 mg/kg/day divided q4-6h) **AND** [gentamicin 7.5 mg/kg/d IV [q 8h] or rifampin 20 mg/kg/d IV infused once daily over 30 min to 3 hours or rifampin PO [bid] (Max dose 600 mg)]
Yersinia	• Treatment only if ill, persistent diarrhea or thalassemia. *Septra* or cefixime PO (pg 84,85) **OR** gentamicin 7.5 mg/kg/d IV (tid)

Common Oral Antimicrobial Doses and Mixtures

Antimicrobial	Formulations	Dose (Frequency) [1]
acyclovir	200,400, 800, 200 mg/5 ml	See infections pg 77-83
albendazole (*Albenza*)	200 mg	See infection (max 400/d)
amoxicillin (*Amoxil*)	Susp: 125, 250 mg/5ml Caps: 125, 250 mg	30-50 mg/kg/day (bid-tid) Max dose 500 mg
amoxicillin/clavulanate (*Augmentin*) [ES]	Susp: 200,400, [600] mg/5ml Tabs: 125, 250, 500 mg	45 mg/kg/day (bid) Max dose 500 mg
ampicillin (*Polycillin*)	Susp: 125, 250 mg/5ml Caps: 250, 500 mg	50-100 mg/kg/day (qid) Max dose 500 mg
azithromycin[2] (*Zithromax*)	Susp: 100, 200, 1000 mg/5ml Caps: 250 mg (max dose 500 mg)	10 mg/kg qd on 1st day, then 5 mg/kg qd x 4d pharyngitis 20mg/kg/d X3d otitis media 30 mg/kg X 1
cefaclor (*Ceclor*) *2nd* generation	Susp: 125, 250 mg/5ml Caps: 250, 500 mg	20-40 mg/kg/day (tid) Max dose 500 mg
cefadroxil (*Duricef*) *1st* generation	Susp: 125,250,500 mg/5ml Cap: 500, Tab: 1000 mg	30 mg/kg/day (bid) Max dose 1000 mg
cefdinir (*Omnicef*) *3rd* generation	Susp: 125 mg/5 ml Cap: 300 mg	14 mg/kg/day (qd-bid) Max daily dose 600 mg
cefixime (*Suprax*) *3rd* generation	Syrup: 100 mg/5ml Tabs: 200, 400 mg	8 mg/kg/day (qd/bid) Max dose 400 mg
cefpodoxime (*Vantin*) *3rd* generation	Susp: 50, 100 mg/5ml Tabs: 100, 200 mg	10 mg/kg/day (bid) Max dose 400 mg
cefprozil (*Cefzil*) *3rd* generation	Susp: 125, 250 mg/5ml Tabs: 250 mg/5ml	15 mg/kg/day (bid) Max dose 500 mg
ceftibuten (*Cedax*) *3rd* generation	Susp: 90, 180 mg/5ml Caps: 400 mg	9 mg/kg/day (qd) Max dose 400 mg
cefuroxime (*Ceftin*) *2nd* generation	Susp: 125 mg/5ml Tabs: 125, 250, 500 mg	15-30 mg/kg/day (bid) Max dose 500 mg
cephalexin (*Keflex*) *1st* generation	Susp: 125, 250 mg/5ml Caps: 250, 500 mg	25-50 mg/kg/day (qid) Max dose 500 mg
clarithromycin (*Biaxin*)	Susp: 125, 250 mg/5 ml Tabs: 250, 500 mg	15 mg/kg/day (bid) Max dose 500 mg
clindamycin (*Cleocin*)	Solution: 75 mg/5ml Cap: 75,150 mg	10-30 mg/kg/day (tid/bid) (30-40 mg/kg/d if DRSP[3]) Max dose 600 mg
dicloxacillin (*Dynapen*)	Susp: 62.5 mg/5ml Caps: 125, 250, 500	25-100 mg/kg/day (qid) Max dose 500 mg
doxycycline(> 8 years) (*Vibramycin*)	Tab/Cap:50,100mg Susp: 25 mg/5 ml, Syrup: 50 mg/5 ml,	2-4 mg/kg/day (bid) Max dose 200 mg/day
erythromycin (*ERYC, EES, E-mycin*)	Susp: 200, 400 mg/5ml Tab: 200(chew),250,400,500	20-50 mg/kg/day (qid) Max dose 500 mg
erythromycin/sulfisox- azole (*Pediazole*)	Susp: 200 mg EM & 600 mg SS per 5ml	20-50 mg/kg/day (qid) Max EM dose 500 mg

[1]*Max Dose = Maximum individual oral dose*, [2]*20mg/kg X 1 dose required for Chlamydia*,
[3] *DRSP – drug resistant S. pneumoniae*

Common Oral Antimicrobial Doses and Mixtures

Antimicrobial	Formulations	Dose (Frequency)
fluconazole (*Diflucan*)	Susp: 10, 40 mg/ml Tabs: 50, 100, 200 mg	3-6 mg/kg/day (qd) Max dose 200 mg
furazolidone (*Furoxone*)	Susp: 50 mg/15ml Tabs: 100 mg	6-8 mg/kg/d X 10 days Max dose 8.8 mg/kg/d
griseofulvin <u>microsize</u> – *Grisactin, Grifulvin V,Fulvicin U/F* <u>ultramicrosize</u> – *Fulvin P/G, Grisactin Ultra*	Susp: 125 mg/5ml Caps: 125, 250 mg Tabs: 125, 165, 250, 330, 500 mg Max dose 1000 mg	10-20 mg/kg/d [bid] micro 5-10 mg/kg/d [qd-bid] ultr <u>tinea corporis</u> X 2 wk <u>tinea pedis/manus</u> X 4 wk <u>tinea capitis</u> X 6 weeks
itraconazole *Sporanox* *Not FDA approved*	Cap: 100 mg, Sol'n 10 mg/ml *Expert recommendations*	3-5 mg/kg/d (see specific infection)
ivermectin (*Stromectol*)	Tab: 3 mg	200 microg/kg/d (see specific infection)
loracarbef (*Lorabid*) 2nd generation	Susp: 100, 200 mg/5ml Caps: 200 mg	15-30 mg/kg/day (bid) Max dose 400 mg
mebendazole (*Vermox*)	Tabs: 100 mg chewable	<u>pinworms</u>: 100 mg X1, repeat in 2 weeks
metronidazole (*Flagyl*)	Tabs: 250, 500 mg	<u>Giardia</u>:15 mg/kg/day (tid) X 7 days
nitrofurantoin (*Macrodantin*)	Susp:25 mg/5ml:Tab: 50,100 mg: Caps: 25, 50, 100 mg	5-7 mg/kg/day (qid) Max dose 100 mg
nystatin (*Mycostatin*)	Susp: 100,000 units/ml Tabs: 500,000 units Max dose 500,000 units	<u>Neo</u>: 1ml q cheek (qid) <u>Child</u>: 500,000 units qid until clear X 48 hrs
penicillin (*Pen-Vee K*)	Susp: 125, 250 per 5 ml Tab: 125, 250, 500 mg	25-50 mg/kg/day (qid) Max dose 500 mg
sulfisoxazole (*Gantrisin*)	Susp: 500 mg/5ml Tab: 500 mg	120-150 mg/kg/day (qid) Max dose 1000 mg
terbinafine (*Lamisil*)	Cap: 250 mg	< 20 kg (62.5 mg), 20-40 kg (125 mg), >40 kg (250)
thiabendazole (*Mintezol*)	Tab: 500 mg Susp: 500 mg/5 ml	44 mg/kg/day Max dose 50 mg/kg/d
trimethoprim / sulfa- methoxazole (*Bactrim, Septra*)	Susp: 40 mg TMP & 200 mg SMX per 5ml Tabs: 80/400, 160/800	6-12 mg of TMP per kg/day (bid) Max dose 160 TMP[1]
vancomycin (*Vancocin*)	Caps: 125, 250	40 mg/kg/d X 7 d Max dose 2000 mg/d

[1]*Higher doses needed for severe UTI, shigella, and pneumocystis infections*

Infective Endocarditis (IE) - Duke Criteria (66% definite/34%possible)

<u>Definitive Criteria</u>: *A – Pathologic Criteria*: Organisms in vegetation, or has embolized, or in intracardiac abscess OR lesions – vegetation or intracardiac abscess confirmed by histology. *B – Clinical criteria* – (1) 2 major or (2) 1 major + 3 minor or (3) 5 minor criteria. <u>Possible criteria</u>: IE findings short of definite but not rejected. <u>Rejected</u>: Firm alternate diagnosis OR, IE symptom resolution OR no evidence of IE at surgery/autopsy with antibiotics ≤ 4 days. **Major Criteria – I Pos. blood culture** for IE <u>IA</u> – typical organisms for IE from 2 blood cultures (BC) – (1) viridans strep, or *S. bovis*, HACEK group, OR (2) community acquired *S. aureus*, or enterococci without primary focus OR <u>IB</u> – persistently + blood culture = recovery of organism consistent with IE from: (1) BC drawn > 12 h apart OR (2) all of 3 or a majority of 4 or more separate BC with 1st & last drawn > 1 h apart. **II Evidence endocardial involvement** – <u>IIA</u> + Echo for IE: (1) oscillating cardiac mass on valve/supporting structures or in regurgitant jet path or on implanted material without alternate explanation OR (2) abscess OR (3) new partial dehiscence prosthetic valve OR <u>IIB</u> – new valvular regurg (not ↑ or change in murmur) **Minor Criteria** – (1) heart condition or IV drugs (2) fever ≥ 38C, (3) vascular Δ – major emboli,septic pulm infarct,mycotic aneurysm, conjunctival bleed, IC bleed, Janeway lesion (4) immune Δ – nephritis, Osler's nodes, Roth spots, RF+, (5) + blood culture (without major criteria) not due to (a) not coag - Staph or(b) bacteria not causing endocarditis or (c) no other evidence of organisms consistent with IE, (6) Echocardiogram ± IE, but no major criteria for IE.

Presenting Features		Underlying Disease-87%		Organisms	
Fever > 38C	97%	VSD	23-28	Strep. viridans	26-32
Immune change[1]	53%	Sys-Pulm shunt	16%	S. aureus	27-29
Malaise/wt loss	39%	Pulm. atresia	14%	Coag neg staph	12-13
Splenomegaly	37-45	Tetrology of F	10-11	Gram neg.	11%
Indwelling cath	32%	Transposition of		S. pneumoniae	7%
Arthralgia	13%	great arteries	8-10%	Candida	3-13%
New murmur	24%	Pulm stenosis	9%	Enterococcus	3-4%
CHF	32%	Prosthetic valve	7%	Strep. bovis	3%
Vasc changes[1]	18%	Aortic stenosis	5-8%	HACEK	
Petechiae	26%	Single ventricle	3-7%	(Haemophilus,	
Dental extract	10%	Coarct aorta	3-10%	Actinobacillus,	
Anemia	68%	MV Prolapse	2-5%	Cardiobacterium,	5%
ESR > 30 mm	68%	Hemodialysis	5%	Eikenella	total
WBC >10,000	54%	Aortic regurg	5%	Kingella)	
Echo +	46-79%	AV canal	5%	Strep agalactiae	2%
Valve or Site		Bicusp aortic vlv	5%	Strep. pyogenes	1%
Mitral	21%	Mitral regurg.	4%	Group C strep	1%
Pulmonary	16%	Tricuspid regurg	4%	Abiotrophia	1%
Mural	16%	Truncus A	4%	Polymicrobial	12%
Triscuspid	10%	Recent cardiac	each	Unknown fungi	1%
Aortic	8%	Cath/surgery	3%	Megasphaeri	1%
Multi, other or ?	29%	Transplant	3%	Culture negative	6-13%

[1] See minor Duke criteria *Pediatr Infect Dis J* 1995;14:1079;*Clin Infect Dis* 1998;27:1451.
Treatment of Infective Endocarditis – See page 78.

Febrile (≥38C) Neonate (≤ 28 days old) Evaluation
• Admit all ≤ 28 days old and perform complete evaluation with IV antibiotic administration (ampicillin 50 mg/kg IV and cefotaxime 50 mg/kg/IV)

Criteria for Outpatient Management of Febrile (≥38C) Infants 29-60 Days Old[1]	
• Well appearing, no underlying illness	• If diarrhea, stool < 5 WBC/HPF and no blood
• WBC < 15,000 cells/mm³	• Normal cerebrospinal fluid
• Serum band to neutrophil ratio < 0.2	• Normal CXR
• Urinalysis < 10 WBC/HPF	• Culture urine, blood, CSF
• Urine with negative gram stain	

[1] Large studies have shown antibiotics are not required if above "Philadelphia" criteria are met and patients have repeat evaluation within 24 hours.

N Engl J Med 1993; 329: 1437; *Pediatrics* 1999; 103: 627.

Fever - Occult Bacteremia (OB)

Overview Primarily has been concern in those with fever ≥ 39C - occurs at all ages & temperatures.	Positive blood culture with no infection and well appearance. Highest risks (age 6-24 mo), WBC > 15,000, absolute neutrophils > 10,000, Yale score > 6. Low risk (0.2%) if viral syndrome (bronchiolitis, croup, stomatitis, varicella). Prior algorithms mandating labs or treatment of well appearing febrile infants are obsolete due to vaccine effectiveness, *S. pneumoniae* meningitis after OB is rare + incompletely prevented with antibiotics, & cost, side effects from treating so many non-bacteremic children.
Haemophilus influenzae type b (HIB)	Mostly eradicated with HIB vaccine. Leads to serious bacterial infection in 25-40%. Positive blood culture mandates reassessment, consideration of spinal tap, IV antibiotics, and admission.
Neisseria meningitidis	Rare cause of OB, in only 0.03% 3-36 months with fever ≥ 39C. 12-46% will see physician & remain undiagnosed at 1st visit. Temperature, WBC & absolute neutrophil count are useless at discriminating febrile viral syndromes from *N. meningitidis* OB. Meningococcus (not OB): 71% have fever > 38C, 4% are < 36.8C, 71% have rash (59% purpura or petechiae, 10% maculopapular, pustular/bullae 1%). Mean WBC 14,000 with 21% < 5,000. 14% have platelets < 100,000 mm³. 55% have meningitis, 11% arthritis, 8% pneumonia. If positive culture or suspicion *N. meningitidis*, admit, IV antibiotics spinal tap. See page 80 for antibiotics and treatment of exposed.
Streptococcus pneumoniae	Prevalence (prior to *S. pneumoniae* vaccine) was 1-2% if 39-39.9C, 2-3% if 40-40.9C, and 4-4½% if ≥ 41C. Only 2% with OB develop meningitis and 10% a serious infection if untreated. With vaccine, prevalence has dropped by 97% in vaccinated with drop also seen in unvaccinated. If positive culture reassess. If appears well, no infection focus, no fever - no treatment needed.

Ann Emerg Med 1998;679; *Arch Pediatr Adolesc Med* 1988;624; *Pediatrics* 1997;100:128; 1999;e20; *Pediatr Infect Dis J* 1989;224 & 2000: 187; *Clin Pediatr* 2001; 583.

Yale Observation Scale (for Infants & Children age 3-36 months)

Observation item	Normal (score 1 point)	Moderate impairment (score 3 points)	Severe impairment (score 5 points)
Quality of cry	strong or none	whimper or sob	weak, moaning, high-pitched, hardly responds
Reaction to parents	cries briefly, no crying, content	cries off and on	persistent cry with little response
State variation	awake, or if asleep wakens quickly	eyes close briefly, awake or wakens with prolonged stimulation	no arousal, falls asleep
Color	pink	pale extremities, acrocyanosis	pale, cyanotic, mottled, or ashen
Hydration	normal skin eyes, mouth	normal skin and eyes, mouth slightly dry	skin doughy/tented, dry mouth, sunken eyes
Response overtures	alert or smiles (consistently)	alert or brief smile	no smile, anxious, dull no alerting to overtures

Total ≤ 10 – 2.7% serious illness (SI), 11-15 – 26% SI, ≥ 16 – 92% SI

Fever and Petechiae Etiology in 190 Children Presenting to a Pediatric ED

Organism identified		No organism found–clinical diagnosis	
Neisseria meningitidis	7%	Viral syndrome	45%
with meningitis	4%	Otitis media	13%
no meningitis	3%	Aseptic meningitis	3%
S. pneumoniae/H flu bacteremia	1%	Pneumonia	3%
Strep. pyogenes pharyngitis	10%	Otitis media with pneumonia	2%
RSV infection	6%	Exudative pharyngitis, partially	1%
Other hemabsorbing virus	6%	treated sepsis or meningitis	each
Enterovirus or rotavirus GI tract	2%	Henoch Schonlein purpura,	0.5%
Enteroviral meningitis	1%	Rocky Mtn Spotted Fever, ALL	each
E. coli urinary tract infection	1%	MMR vaccine reaction	1%

Mandl analyzed 411 consecutive children with fever & petechiae at a pediatric ED and (8) 2% had bacteremia or sepsis with 2 cases each of *N. meningitidis/S. pneumoniae*, 1 Group A strep. sepsis, and 3 with negative cultures. Well appearing children had a 0% (0-3%, 95% confidence interval [CI]) probability of serious infection (SBI), if they had a WBC of 5-15,000 they had a 0% (0-2%, 95% CI) probability of SBI & if no purpura they had a 0% (0-1% 95% CI) probability of SBI. *Baker Pediatrics* 1989; 84: 1051; Mandl *J Pediatr* 1997; 131: 398.

Bacterial Meningitis - Clinical Features

History[1]	Frequency	Exam[1]	Frequency	Nuchal rigidity[2]	
History fever	• 95%	Temp ≥38.3C	• 59-77%	Age	Frequency
Lethargy or		Altered LOC	• 53-78%	0-6 months	27%
Irritability	• 87-95%	ENT infection	• 22-44%	7-12 months	71%
Vomiting	• 54-71%	Focal deficit	• 5-6%	13-18 months	87%
URI	• 46-55%			> 18 months	95%

[1]*Ann Emerg Med* 1992;21:146. [2]*Ann Emerg Med* 1992;21:911.

Tick Borne Disease

Ehrlichiosis

	Features in Pediatric HME	
Human monocytic & granulocytic ehrlichiosis (HME & HGE) = febrile illnesses due to rickettsia transmitted by Lone Star or wood tick esp. in SE, southcentral, midwest US. 90% April-Sept. Deer livestock - hosts. Incubation is 12-14 d. Diagnose - Wright stain, antibody titer (*CDC requires compatible Hx + ≥1:64 titer or 4 X change acute & convalescent titers*). <u>Treatment</u> – doxycycline (4 mg/kg/day divided bid [max 100 mg/dose] X 7-10 d if > 8 y. Doxycycline or chloramphenicol if ≤ 8y.	• Fever	100%
	• Known tick bite	82%
	• Headache/myalgia	63%
	• ↑ Liver/Spleen	41%
	• Rash trunk+extremity macule/papule/petech	66%
	• ↑ LFT	89%
	• ↓ platelets	82%
	• ↓WBC/lymphocytes	69/80
	• ↓Sodium	65%
	• Anemia	39%

Pediatrics 1997; 100: e10; *J Pediatr* 1997; 131: 184.

Lyme Disease

	Features in Children	
Inflammatory disease vs multiple organs due to spirochete (*Borrelia burgdorferi*) transmitted by ticks (deer tick). Disease can be (1) early local 1-2 weeks - (ECM/erythema chronicum migrans) red macule or papule-expands to large size (mean 16 cm in adults) resolves over weeks. (2) early disseminated 2-12 weeks - carditis, early arthritis (mean 2.4 large joints; knee > ankle; 2 to 100,000 cells/mm³, esp eosinophils), meningitis, multiple EM lesions. (3) chronic arthritis or neuro deterioration. Diagnose by ELISA or IFA followed by more specific West. immunoblot if equivocal or + 1st test. <u>Treatment</u> – see page 79.	• ECM rash esp. at skin crease (mean adult size 16 cm)	68%
	• Flu like symptoms	64%
	• Arthritis/arthralgia (40% > 1 joint)	59%
	• Known tick bite	49%
	• ECG changes esp. 1st degree AVblock	29%
	• Bell's palsy (7th CN)	14%
	• Aseptic meningitis	4%
	• Myelitis/neuropathy	1%

J Pediatr Orthop 1994;238. *Pediatr Emerg Care* 1991;334; *Pediatr Infect Dis J* 1990;10.

Rocky Mountain Spotted Fever

	Features in Children
RMSF - vasculitis due to *R. rickettsii* - South Atlantic US. Wood & dog tick transmit. 90% April to September with 2/3 < 15 y. Incubation is 2-12 days. Tests - not positive until 6-10 d. Weil Felix test = inaccurate, no longer used to diagnose. <u>Treatment</u> – Mortality is rare if treat before 5th day of illness, therefore, observe in 1st 2-4 days if uncertain diagnosis & well appearing. Use doxycycline > 8 y, while risk/benefits of doxycycline or chloramphenicol or fluoroquinolone must be considered if ≤ 8y. See pg 82 for dose	• Headache/Myalgias/fever
	• Rash (95%) – periph.onset
	• Palm/sole rash (50-75%)
	• Seizures/Meningismus
	• DIC/shock
	• WBC count –normal or ↓
	• ↓Platelets, ↓ Hb,
	• ↓ Sodium, ↑ BUN, ↑ LFTs
	• Biopsy immunohistology IFA 70% sensitive/100% specific
	• ELISA/IF antibody tests +

www.cdc.gov; *Pediatr Rev* 1998; 171; *Pediatr Infect Dis J* 1999; 539.

Tick Bite –Single doxycycline dose (↑ Lyme endemic area) ↓'d erythema migrans from 3.2% to 0.4%. Dose 3.0 mg/kg PO (maximum 200 mg). Risks, benefits, side effects esp. in those ≤ 8 years must be considered. *N Engl J Med 2001; 345: 79.*

Tick Paralysis –Toxin produced by Rocky Mtn wood tick > dog tick. Exposure to tick occurs 5-10 days prior to symptoms. In US, 82% are < 8 years old. Rapid ascending paralysis over 12-36 hours. Bulbar (eye muscle) involved early. 50% have parasthesias - most - most = normal sensory exam. In 1 series all cases occurred from March to June. Tick is often hidden on body (esp. hairline/scalp). Removal of tick is curative although Australian form of disease may worsen over ≥ 48 hours after removal and may be amenable to anti-toxin. *Clin Infect Dis 1999; 29: 1435.*

Tick Removal - Procedure

- Apply gloves ± inject small wheal of lidocaine + epi. directly beneath tick.
- Applying petroleum jelly, alcohol, fingernail polish or hot match to underside of tick may cause regurgitation (of organisms) and **should be avoided**.
- Using blunt tweezers, grasp the tick as close as possible to the skin.
- Pull slowly in a firm perpendicular direction away from the skin.
- Do not squeeze the tick and do not rotate as pulling away from skin.
- Cleanse area thoroughly after procedure with disinfectant.
- Person performing procedure should thoroughly wash hands afterwards.
- Place tick into alcohol or flush down toilet.

Respiratory Tract Infections

CDC Recommendations for Treating Acute Otitis Media (AOM)

	No Antibiotics (Abx) prior month[1]	Antibiotics in prior month
Day 0	amoxicillin 40-45 mg/kg or ↑ dose[2] amoxicillin 80-90 mg/kg	↑ dose amoxicillin or *Augmentin* 80-90 mg/kg, cefuroxime[2]
Day 3 Rx failure	↑ dose amoxicillin/*Augmentin* 80-90 mg/kg, cefuroxime[3], ceftriaxone IM qd X 3 d (or recheck 48 h after 1st dose)	ceftriaxone IM qd X 3 days (or recheck for improvement 48 h after 1st dose), clindamycin[4], tympanocentesis
Day 10-28 Rx failure	Same as day 3	↑ dose *Augmentin* 80-90 mg/kg, cefuroxime[3], ceftriaxone IM X 3 days, or tympanocentesis

[1] duration of therapy (Rx) – if < 2 years or chronic/recurrent AOM, treat for 10 days, if > 2 years + uncomplicated AOM, acceptable options: (1) observe for symptom resolution with Abx given at 72 hours if still symptomatic (↓ Abx use by 75%), or (2) 5-7 day Abx regimen
[2] use ↑dose if drug resistant *S. pneumoniae* (DRSP) likely (day care, Abx use prior mo);
[3] cefdinir may be substituted for cefuroxime in algorithm
[4] clindamycin has adequate activity against DRSP but not for *H. influenzae*, or *M. catarrhalis*.
[5] *Pediazole, Septra* & erythromycin are alternatives in penicillin/cephalosporin allergic patients, however 30-40% of *S. pneumoniae* strains are not susceptible to these agents & these Abx are not as effective as β lactams for AOM due to *H. influenzae*. Azithromycin and clarithromycin have similar clinical efficacy compared to high dose *Augmentin*; however, with less side effects and similar overall cure rates.

Ped Infect Dis J 1999; 1 & 2000; 938; Ann EM 2002;34:413. Pediatrics 2001; 108: 239

CDC/AAP Guidelines for Judicious Use of
Antibiotics (Abx) in Pediatric Respiratory Infections

Common cold	• Do not give antibiotics for the common cold. • Mucopurulent rhinitis is not indication for Abx unless it lasts > 10-14 days.
Acute Otitis Media (AOM) & Otitis Media with Effusion (OME)	• Diagnosis of AOM requires documented middle ear effusion and signs or symptoms of acute local or systemic illness. • Uncomplicated AOM may be treated with 5-7 days of Abx if > 2 years old. • Persistent effusion after AOM therapy is expected and does not need Abx • Abx are not indicated for OME unless effusion persists for ≥ 3 months • Abx prophylaxis should be reserved for control of recurrent AOM (defined as ≥ 3 distinct/well documented episodes in 6 mo or ≥ 4 in 12 months)
Pharyngitis	• Diagnosis of group A strep pharyngitis should be based on results of appropriate lab tests in conjunction with clinical epidemiologic findings. • Abx should not be given to a child with pharyngitis in the absence of diagnosed group A strep or other bacterial infection. • A penicillin is drug of choice for group A strep. pharyngitis
Sinusitis	(Includes 2001 AAP Clinical Practice Guideline – *Pediatrics* 2001; 108:798) • Clinical diagnosis of bacterial sinusitis requires prolonged nonspecific upper respiratory signs and symptoms (e.g. rhinosinusitis/cough > 10-14 d) or more severe features (temp ≥ 39C, facial swelling or pain). • Radiographs are only indicated if recurrence, complications suspected, or when the diagnosis is unclear (common cold causes Xray changes). CT should be reserved for patients in whom surgery is being considered. • See CDC antibiotic recommendations page 82.

Pediatr Infect Dis J 1999; 19: 907; *Pediatrics* 2001; 108: 798.

Clinical Scoring for Group A Streptococcal Pharyngitis

		Total	PPV[1]
Fever > 38.3C (101F)	*Each of 6 features*	1	0%
Age 5-15 years	*is worth one point*	2 or 3	20%
Nov-May presentation	*(mnemonic = FANCUP)*	4	42%
Cervical adenopathy		5	63%
URI absent (i.e., cough, rhinorrhea, congestion)		6	75%
Pharyngitis (i.e., tonsillar erythema, hypertrophy, or exudate)			

[1]Positive predictive value for Group A streptococcus.

Pediatr Emerg Care 1998;14:109.

Urinary Tract Infections (UTI)

Organisms in neonates: E coli 74%, klebsiella 7%, pseudomonas 7%, proteus 4%. In older infants/children: E coli is most common. Proteus and pseudomonas are more common if hospitalized, recurrent UTI, or male.	Age	UTI Risk[1]
	0-2 months	7.5%
	2-24 months	4.1%
	2-5 years	1.7%

[1]If fever present

Risk factors and Symptoms of UTI in Febrile Infants and Children < 3 years old	Most Common UTI Symptoms		Risk of UTI if Feature Present	
	irritability	80%	female > 39 C	8.8%
	poor feeding	65%	fever without source	7.5%
	vomiting/diarrhea	30-40%	fever + otitis media	3.5%
	URI symptoms	10-20%	fever + major source	1.5%

Pediatr Ann 1993; 505. J Pediatr 1993; 123: 17

Diagnosis: 93% of + bag UA cultures are contaminants, therefore catheter specimen is preferred. Nitrate + = E coli, proteus, klebsiella, enterobacter, salmonella; (not S. saprophyticus, pseudomonas, enterococcus). A UA is insensitive for UTI; culture if < 3-5y.

Predictive Value of Urinalysis in Detecting UTI

Urinalysis feature	Sensitivity	Negative predictive value
Any WBC/high power field (hpf)	77%	97%
≥ 5 WBC/hpf	43-84%	90-98%
Any bacteria	86-93%	99%
+ leuk esterase,nitrate,or ≥ 5WBC/hpf	75-98%	85-99%
Positive gram stain for bacteria	94-99%	99%

Pediatrics 1999; 103; e54; Pediatr Infect Dis J 2001; 20: 40.

Management Options for Urinary Tract Infection _Pediatrics 1999; 103: 843._

Admit	• ≤ 3 months old, obstruction, high grade reflux, dehydration, vomiting, toxicity, nephrolithiasis, or immunocompromised
IV antibiotics	• gentamicin 7.5 mg/kg/d IV divided q 8h + ampicillin 100 mg/kg/d IV divide q 12h (esp. if gram positive bacteria) **OR** • ceftriaxone 75 mg/kg/d IV (do not use < 28 days old) **OR** • cefotaxime 150 mg/kg/d IV divided q 6-8 h
Oral Antibiotics	• cefixime, _Septra, Augmentin,_ cephalexin. Treat for 14 days if fever or toxic, 7-14 days if no fever and no toxicity. See page 84,85 for doses.
Urinary Tract Evaluation	• No clinical response within 1st 48 h: immediate urinary tract ultrasound (to exclude abscess or obstruction) + voiding cysto-urethrogram (VCUG) or radionuclide cystography (RNC) at earliest convenience. VCUG preferred in males as it assesses urethra for posterior valves. • If nontoxic or doing well, VCUG or RNC at earliest convenience • Continue antibiotics while awaiting above study • Radionuclide renal scans/DMSA and CT will identify acute changes from pyelonephritis or renal scarring. Their exact role in aiding management of a child with UTI is still undefined.

Guidelines for Pediatric Intensive Care Unit Admission

General	• Severe, potentially life-threatening, unstable disorders
Cardiovascular	• Post CPR, shock, or unstable congestive heart failure • Dysrhythmias (life threatening), temporary pacing • Congenital heart disease with unstable status • Arterial, central venous, pulmonary artery monitoring
Endocrine & Metabolic	• Severe DKA requiring therapy exceeding institutional patient care unit guidelines • Severe electrolyte △ (e.g. ↑K requiring monitoring or acute intervention, severe ↑ or ↓ Na/Ca/glucose) • Monitoring required for complex interventions to treat fluid balance or severe acidosis (e.g. $NaHCO_3$) • Inborn errors of metabolism with possible deterioration requiring respiratory support, dialysis, ↑ICP, BP support
Gastroenterology	• Severe bleed, post endoscopy for FB removal, liver failure with coma/BP/respiratory instability
Hematology & Oncology	• Exchange transfusion, severe coagulopathy, severe anemia with BP/respiratory compromise, sickle cell complication (acute chest syndrome, aplastic crisis, stroke) • Initiated chemo. with anticipated tumor lysis syndrome • Tumors or masses compressing vessels, organs, airway • Plasmapheresis/leukapheresis and unstable
Multi-system	• Toxic ingestion with decompensation potential • Multiorgan dysfunction syndrome, burn > 10% surface • Environmental (hypo/hyperthermia, electrical injury)
Neurologic	• Unresponsive seizures,↓LOC with possible deterioration • Post-neurosurgery requiring invasive monitor/observation, placement of external ventricular drainage device • CNS inflammation with possible neurologic depression, metabolic or hormonal abnormality, CV instability, ↑ICP • Preop neurosurgical with deterioration, any ↑ICP • Spinal cord compression or impending compression • Progressive neuromuscular dysfunction requiring support
Renal	• Acute renal failure, acute rhabdomyolysis/renal insuff. • Requires acute hemodialysis, peritoneal dialysis, or continuous renal replacement therapy and unstable
Respiratory	• Endotracheal intubation or potential for ventilator • Rapidly progressive up/low airway disease/failure • Requires ≥ 50 %FiO2, newly placed tracheostomy • Inhaled nebulizer/meds above ability of general unit
Surgical	• Select postop – cardiovascular, thoracic, neurosurg, ENT, ortho or spine, general surg, transplant, major blood loss • Major trauma with/without instability

Pediatric Section Task Force, Society of Crit Care Med. *Crit Care Med* 1999; 27: 843.

Kawasaki's Disease

Overview: Kawasaki's disease is an acute vasculitis of unknown origin. Kawasaki's leads to cardiac complications in 25% of cases, and is the #1 acquired heart disease in children. The earliest sign is high fever (often ≥ 40ºC) for up to 10 days. Small and medium arteries are affected throughout body, with infiltration & destruction of intima & media by macrophages, lymphocytes, & mast cells.	**Phases of Kawasaki's Disease** • *Acute phase* (0-2 weeks from onset) Sudden fever, rash, conjunctivitis, lymphadenopathy, mucosal changes, and/or myocarditis • *Subacute phase* (2-8 weeks) Arthritis, epidermal desquamation (beginning periungually), possibility of cardiac thrombi/aneurysm forming • *Convalescent phase* (up to 2 years) - Risk of coronary aneurysm

Diagnostic Criteria[1]

Fever lasting at least 5 days without other source, and at least 4 of the following:
- Bilateral conjunctival injection (painless, and without exudate)
- Mucous membrane changes (e.g., injected pharynx, strawberry tongue, or redness, fissuring, and crusting of lips)
- Edema or erythema of palms or soles (desquamation in convalescent phase)
- Rash (polymorphous and truncal)
- Cervical adenopathy, with at least one node > 1.5 cm

[1]Other *nondiagnostic* features: sleep disturbances (90%), urethritis and sterile pyuria (75%), uveitis/iritis (80%) arthralgias/arthritis (~30%), or hemolytic uremic syndrome (rare)

Diagnostic Tests

- Platelet count > 1 million, during (subacute) thrombosis stage, normal acutely
- Leukocytosis, with left shift, mild hemolytic anemia, CRP and ESR elevation
- Urine - Moderate pyuria, occasional bilirubinuria due to gallbladder hydrops
- CXR – Cardiomegaly in up to 30%
- ECG – 1st week: low voltage, ST depression, 2nd-3rd week: PR and QT prolongation, ST elevation

Evaluation and treatment

- Gamma globulin: Administer 2 grams/kg IV over 8-12 h as a single infusion.
- Aspirin: 80-100 mg/kg/day PO divided qid until 14th day of illness, then 3-5 mg/kg PO qd until 6-8 weeks after onset. If coronary artery aneurysm is evident on echocardiogram, continuation of ASA beyond 8 weeks may be indicated.
- Obtain echocardiogram on presentation. Repeat 14, 21 & 60 days after onset.

MA	NH₄	Glu	Specific Inborn Errors of Metabolism[1]
↔	↔	↔	Nonketotic hyperglycinemia
↔	↑	↔	**Citrulline normal** (transient hyperammonemia of newborn or HHH [hyperornithinemia, hyperammoniemia, & homocitrullinuria]); **Urea cycle disorders** *low citrulline* (↓ ornithine transcarbamylase or ↓ carbamyl phosphate synthetase), *mild ↑ citrulline* (↓ argininosuccinate lyase), *↑ citrulline* (citrullinemia)
↑	↑	↓	**Fatty acid oxidation** - carnitine deficiency, medium/long/short chain CoA dehydrogenase **Organic acidemia** - dicarboxylic aciduria, glutaric acidemia type II (K), methylmalonic acidemia (K,L), propionic acidemia (K,L), congenital lactic acidosis (K,L)
↑	↑	↔	Periodic hyperlysinemia, **Organic acidemia**: ↓ ketothiolase
↑	↑	↑	**Organic acidemias**: isovaleric acidemia (K,L), methylmalonic acidemia (K,L), propionic acidemia (K,L)
↑	↔	↔	**Organic acidemia**: isovaleric acidemia
↑	↔	↓	**Carbohydrate metabolism**: fructose 1,6 diphosphatase deficient (L), **Glycogen storage type** I,III (K), **Amino aciduria**: maple syrup urine disease (early onset), glutaric aciduria type I

[1]**MA**: ↑ metabolic acidosis with anion gap vs. ↔ no metabolic acidosis <u>NH₄</u>: ↑ hyperammonemia vs. ↔ normal ammonia; <u>Glu</u>: ↑ hyperglycemia vs. ↔ normoglycemia vs ↓ hypoglycemia; <u>K</u> – ketonuria, <u>L</u> – lactic acidosis

Typical Presentations

Hyperammonia –neonatal catastrophe, seizures, ↓ feed, coma, loss of tone, recurrent coma, vomiting, lethargy after high protein food, FTT, recurrent vomiting, ataxia, improves with IV fluids or recurrent coma , mental retardation, growth failure

Organic Acidurias –neonatal catastrophe, recurrent coma, mental retardation, growth failure, liver failure after virus, smells (e.g. maple syrup, sweaty sock, musty)

Management

Evaluation	• Blood – glucose, CBC, electrolytes, Ca, LFTs, bilirubin, NH₄, quantitative amino acids, lactate, pyruvate, carnitine, fatty acids • Urine – ketone bodies, reducing substances, protein, quantitative amino acids, organic acids, galactose • CSF- glucose, protein, cell count, microscopy, lactate, amino acids
Catabolism	• Reverse catabolism with IV fluids plus dextrose
Precipitant	• Search for/treat precipitant (e.g. infection) & coexisting hypoglycemia
Acidosis	• Liberal NaHCO₃ due to ongoing acid production + dialysis • If organic acidemia, B12 1 mg IM (methylmalonic acidemia) + Biotin 10 mg PO or NG (multiple carboxylase deficiency), thiamine 25-100 mg PO (MSUD), folic acid 1-5 mg PO (methylmalonic acidemia with homocystinuria), vitamin C & K (primary lactic acidosis due to electron transport defect) glycine (isovaleric acidemia) & carnitine (↓carnitine)
Ammonia	• Dialysis, lactulose. If urea cycle defect (NH₄ with no acids) (1) arginine HCl 6 ml/kg of 10% solution IV over 90 min (citrullinemia, argininosuccinic aciduria), (2) sodium benzoate (OTC/CPS deficiency)

Renal Disorders

Urinalysis: False + dipstick for blood occur with UTI's, betadine, ascorbic acid. RBC casts or dysmorphic RBC's suggest glomerular disease. Infants < 3 months old cannot concentrate urine well, therefore, specific gravity is unreliable at this age.

Causes of Red Urine

Hematuria, alcaptonuria, bilirubinemia, phenazopyridine, phenothiazines, ibuprofen, L-dopa, phenolphthalein, methyldopa, adriamycin, deferoxamine, phenytoin, quinine, sulfa, chloroform, naphthalene, oxalic acid, anilines, food color, beets, blueberries, rhubarb, fava beans, hemoglobinuria or myoglobinuria (Heme + dipstick with no RBC's), porphyrins, red diaper syndrome (*Serratia*), tyrosinosis.

Differential Diagnosis of Hematuria (see page 97 for evaluation)

- *Extrarenal disorders:* coagulation disorders, salicylates, sickle cell disease/trait
- *Renal extraglomerular:* hemorrhagic cystitis, trauma, nephrolithiasis, familial hypercalciuria, nephritis, hydronephrosis, polycystic kidneys, renal vein thrombosis, papillary necrosis, hemangiomas, tumor (e.g., Wilm's), foreign body, posterior urethral valves, ureteropelvic junction obstruction, renal tuberculosis.
- *Renal glomerular:* glomerulonephritis, IgA nephropathy, Alport's syndrome, exercise, familial benign hematuria, focal glomerulosclerosis.
- *Systemic:* allergy, hepatitis B antigenemia, endocarditis, cardiac shunt or valve, Henoch-Schonlein purpura, hemolytic uremic syndrome, polyarteritis.

Normal Bladder Volume and Normal Plasma Creatinine (PCr)

Bladder volume Estimate	• < 1 year old: weight (kg) X 10 ml • > 1 year old: (age in years + 2) X 30 ml
Plasma Creatinine Estimate	• Males: PCr (mg/dl) = 0.35 + (0.025 x age in years) • Females: PCr (mg/dl) = 0.35 + (0.018 x age in years)

Differentiating Between Causes of Renal Failure

Test	Pre-renal	Renal	Post-renal
Urine sodium	< 20	> 40	> 40
Fractional excretion of sodium[1]	< 1	> 2	> 2
Renal failure index[2]	< 1	> 2	> 2
Urine osmolality	> 500	< 300	< 400
Urine/serum creatinine ratio	> 40	< 20	< 20
Serum BUN/creatinine ratio	> 20	< 10-20	< 10-20
Renal size by ultrasound	normal	normal	normal or ↑
Radionuclide renal scan	↓uptake ↓excretion	uptake OK ↓excretion	uptake OK ↓excretion

[1] FE_{Na} = 100 x (urine Na^+/plasma Na^+) / (urine creatinine/plasma creatinine)
   Normal FE_{Na} is 1-2%, except under 2 months when FE_{Na} up may be to 5%.
[2] RFI = (urine Na^+) / (urine creatinine / serum creatinine)

Evaluation of Atraumatic Microscopic Hematuria[1]

assuming no vaginal, GI, urethral prolapse, hematologic disease, or UTI source
(See page 169, 170 for Evaluation of Traumatic Hematuria)

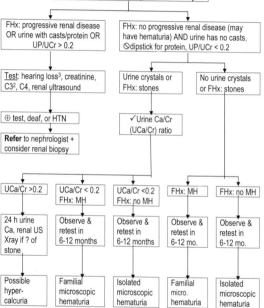

[1] FHx – family history, UP – urine protein, UCr – urine creatinine, UCa – urine calcium,
HTN – hypertension, Ca – calcium, US – ultrasound

[2] Depressed C3/4 associated with postinfectious glomerulonephritis, SLE, membrano-
proliferative glomerulonephritis, endocarditis, shunt nephritis, Hep B, HIV.

[3] e.g. Alport's syndrome

Pediatrics 1998; 102: e42.

Neurology

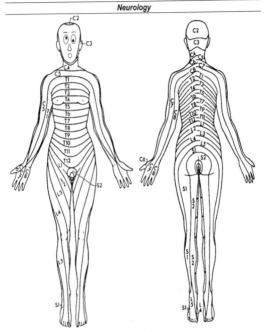

Motor level	Motor function
C4	spontaneous breathing
C5	shoulder shrug
C6	elbow flexion
C7	elbow extension
C8/T1	finger flexion
T1-T12	intercostal and abdominal muscles

Motor level	Motor function
L1/L2	hip flexion
L3	hip adduction
L4	hip abduction
L5	great toe dorsiflexion
S1/S2	foot plantar flexion
S2-S4	rectal tone

Assessment of Coma and Altered Level of Consciousness

Trauma or tumor	**A**buse or alcohol	_Differential_
Infection/Intussusception	**E**ncephalopathy/Endocrine	_Diagnosis of_
Poisons	**I**nsulin/hypoglycemia	_Coma & ALOC_
Sepsis, Seizure, Shock	or metabolic error	
	Opiates	mnemonic
	Uremia	**TIPS-AEIOU**

	Infant	Child	Adolescent
Common Causes of Altered Mental Status by Age	Infection	Ingestion	Ingestion
	Metabolic (inborn or acquired disorder)	Infection	Trauma
		Intussusception	Poison
	Abuse	Seizure/abuse	Psychogenic

Treatment of Infant/Child with an Altered Mental Status

- Assess airway and breathing (immobilizing cervical spine if possible trauma).
- Consider endotracheal intubation if poor or labored respiratory effort, diminished airway reflexes, suspicion of elevated ICP, or severe hypoxemia.
- Assess pulse oximetry and administer 100% oxygen.
- Obtain rapid glucose measurement or administer glucose (dosage, page 38).
- Consider naloxone 0.1 mg/kg.
- Measure child's length to facilitate dosing and sizing of equipment (see page 5).
- Complete vital signs: temp, respirations, pulse, & BP. Perform complete exam.
- Direct further evaluation based on above measures, and history + examination.

Normal Neonatal/Infant Reflexes Appearance/Disappearance

Reflex (description)	Appears	Disappears
Moro - lift head 30° and let fall to neutral. A positive test = arm extension and abduction, then arm adduction	Birth	1-3 months
Palmar grasp - object in hand causes flexion/grasping	Birth	4 months
Root response - stroking cheek causes mouth to turn in direction of stimulus	Birth	3-4 months
Tonic neck - turn head to side while child is supine, with ipsilateral arm & leg extending and opposite arm/leg flexing. Normal infant tries to break reflex position.	Birth	5-6 months
+ _Babinski_ - stroking lateral border of sole, to big toe. A positive reflex causes big toe dorsiflexion, and fanning of other toes	Birth	1-2 years

Most Common Etiologies	Viral illness	39%	Strep throat	5%
of Headache in Children	Sinusitis	16%	Tension	5%
Presenting to a Pediatric	Migraine	16%	Other disease	8%
Emergency Department	Post-trauma	7%	Serious CNS	
Pediatr Emerg Care 1997;13:1.	Viral meningitis	5%	disorders[1]	7%

[1] includes 5% viral meningitis, and < 0.3% each of bleed, tumor, hydrocephalus

---

Seizures and Status Epilepticus

Neonatal Seizures

Seizure type	Clinical Manifestations
Subtle	Oral-buccal-lingual movements; ocular movements
	Stereotypic pedaling/swimming/stepping
	Autonomic dysfunction - abnormal HR, BP or oxygenation
	(Apnea rarely occurs without other manifestations of seizure)
Clonic	Rhythmic, slow jerking; focal or multifocal
	Facial, extremity or axial involvement
Tonic	Sustained limb posturing; may be focal or generalized
	Asymmetric position of trunk/neck
Myoclonic	Rapid isolated jerks; Generalized, multifocal or focal
	Limb or trunk involvement

Pediatr in Review 2000; 21: 117.

Neonatal Seizure Mimics

Movement Disorder	Clinical Manifestations
Jitteriness	• Occurs spontaneously or due to stimulus
	• Flexion and extension are equivalent
	• Repositioning/flexion of extremity is diminished
	• No abnormal eye movements
Benign neonatal sleep myoclonus	• Bi or unilateral, may be synchronous or asynchronous
	• Occurs during sleep and is not due to stimulus
Stimulus-evoked myoclonus	• Focal or generalized, severe CNS dysfunction
	• EEG may show cortical spike-wave discharge
Hyperekplexia (stiff-man syndrome)	• Inherited, apnea and bradycardia may occur
	• Generalized myoclonus with hyperactivity after startle
	• Severe hypertonia responsive to benzodiazepines

Differentiation of	Absence Seizure	Nonepileptic Staring
Absence Seizures	Limb twitching	Play not interrupted
from	Upward eye movement	Respond to touch
Nonepileptic	Urinary incontinence	Body rocking
Staring		Teacher/health worker 1st saw

J Pediatr 1998; 133: 660

Most Common Seizure Etiology by Age

Day 1	
Hypoxia (perinatal-intrauterine)	Infection (group B streptococcus, E. coli)
Birth trauma (subarachnoid, subdural)	Drugs (e.g. cocaine), low pyridoxine
↑ or ↓ glucose, ↓ calcium	Anesthetic injection

Days 2 - 3	
Hypoxia, Infection, Drug withdrawal	Developmental malformations
Hyponatremia, Hypernatremia	Intracranial hemorrhage
Hypoglycemia, Hypocalcemia (day 3-14)	Inborn errors of metabolism (page 95)

Days 4 – 6 Months	
Infection	Developmental malformations
Hypocalcemia (esp. days 3-14)	Drug withdrawal (esp. narcotics)
Hyperphosphatemia	Inborn errors of metabolism (days 4-14)
Hyponatremia	aminoaciduria, organic aciduria, urea cycle

6 months – 3 Years	
Febrile seizures, Birth injury	Trauma, metabolic disorder
Infection, or Toxin	Cerebral degeneration

> 3 Years	
Idiopathic, Infection, Trauma	Cerebral degeneration

Practice Parameter: Evaluation of 1st Nonfebrile Seizure > 1 Month Old

Lab tests[1]	• Order labs (CBC, glucose, electrolytes) based on clinical circumstances (e.g. vomiting, diarrhea, dehydration, failure to return to baselines status). ↓Na & ↓Ca (most common unrecognized △) are rare - more common if ≤ 6 months. • Consider toxicology screen if any question of exposure[3]
Lumbar puncture[1]	• Perform only if suspect CNS infection/Subarachnoid bleed
EEG[2]	• Perform on all first time non-febrile seizures
Neuroimaging[1] MRI is preferred to CT for identifying etiology, CT is more available acutely & excludes life threats - bleed or mass effect	• Perform emergent neuroimaging if postictal focal deficits or altered mental status does not resolve rapidly • Nonurgent MRI should be seriously considered in any child with (1) significant cognitive or motor impairment of unknown etiology, (2) abnormal exam, (3) focal seizure without secondary generalization, (4) EEG that does not represent a benign partial epilepsy of childhood or primary generalized epilepsy or (5) age ≤ 1 year

[1]Options – not necessary in all, [2]Standard – recommended in all,
[3]See page 141 for drugs causing seizures

Seizure Mimics in Infants, Children, & Adolescents

Infant	Child[1]	Adolescent[1]
jitteriness (withdrawal), tremor	breath holding	vagal, orthostasis
apnea (> 20 sec with cyanosis)	cough syncope	migraine
micturitional shivering	night tremor, night terror	hyperventilation
dysrhythmia	migraine	pseudoseizures
Sandifer syndrome (GE reflux)	tics	hysteria

[1]in general patients have precipitant, premonitory symptoms, and are not post-ictal

Febrile seizures – Seizure occurring between 6 months and 5 years, associated with fever, but without evidence of intracranial infection or defined cause.
Simple febrile seizures generalized, < 15 min, only 1 seizure. 25-33% reoccur. Recurrence is more common if 1st degree relative with afebrile or febrile seizures, complex features, age < 1 y (50% recurrence) or lower temp at onset (temp 101 – 35%; 102 – 30%, 103 – 26%, 104 – 20%, and 105 – 13% recurrence). Manage - consists of identify/treat cause of the fever. ±LP if unreliable exam (on antibiotics, very young). **Complex febrile seizure** - > 15 min, focal, > 1 in 24 h, abnormal neuro. exam after seizure. Consider complete work up CT, LP & labs, EEG.

Most Common Etiologies of Status Epilepticus in Children < 16 years Old			
	Fever/Infection	36%	Anoxia	5%
	Med Change	20%	Infection	5%
	Unknown	9%	Trauma	4%
	Metabolic	8%	CVA[1]	3%
Pediatr Emerg Care 1999;15:119.	Congenital	7%	Ethanol/drugs	2%

[1] CVA – cerebrovascular accident

Management of Status Epilepticus

- Protect airway, administer O_2, start IV, cardiac monitor, pulse oximeter. Perform stat bedside glucose test and send electrolytes and drug levels.
- Administer IV glucose (10 ml/kg of D_{10}W if a neonate, 4 ml/kg of D_{25}W if <2 y, 2 ml/kg of D_{50}W if >2 y), & pyridoxine 50-100 mg IV if neonate.
- Intravenous drug therapy as per table. If 1st drug is unsuccessful, try another agent (sequence A,B,C,D). If unsuccessful, consider general anesthesia.
- Treat fever/infection and correct sodium, calcium, or magnesium abnormalities.

Intravenous Drug Therapy for Status Epilepticus (A - D preferred order)

	Drug	Dose & route	Maximum rate	Special features
A	lorazepam	0.05-0.15 mg/kg IV	<0.5-1 mg/min	may repeat q5 min x2
	or diazepam	0.2-0.3 mg/kg IV	<1.0 mg/min	may repeat q5 min x2
	or diazepam	0.5 mg/kg PR	--	may repeat ½ dose x1
B	fosphenytoinPE[1]	15-18 mg/kg IV	< 2 mg/kg/min	monitor closely
	or phenytoin	15-18 mg/kg IV	< 0.5 mg/kg/min	monitor closely
C	phenobarbital[2]	15-20 mg/kg IV	< 1.0 mg/kg/min	monitor closely
D	midazolam **or**	0.2 mg/kg IV or IM		drip at 1-10 microg/kg/min
	pentobarbital (coma)[3]	10-15 mg/kg IV load 0.5-3.0 mg/kg/h	over 10-30 min & < 50 mg/min	intubation required; vasopressors prn

[1] PE–phenytoin equivalents: all doses and rates are in phenytoin equivalents,
[2] may ↑ to total 40 mg/kg or 1 g max, [3]attach EEG if possible

Shunts (Cerebrospinal Shunt Infection and Malfunction)

CSF Shunt Obstruction – Predictive Score

Early Presenters (within 5 months of surgery)		Late Presenters (> 9 months to 2 years since surgery)	
Clinical Feature	Points	Clinical Feature	Points
Fluid tracking around shunt	1	Nausea & vomiting	1
Headache	1	Loss of developmental milestones	1
Irritability	1	↑ Head circumference	1
Fever	1	Fluid tracking around shunt	1
Bulging fontanelle	2	↓ Level of consciousness	3
Erythema at surgery site	3		
↓ Level of consciousness	3		
Early shunt score (total points above)	Shunt Failure Probability	Late shunt score (total points above)	Shunt Failure Probability
0 points	4%	0 points	8%
1 point	50%	1 point	38%
2 points	75%	≥ 2 points	100%
≥ 3 points	100%		

Other features (not found to be independent predictors of shunt failure) include inability to depress or refill CSF reservoir, papilledema, cranial nerve palsy, abd. pain/mass, meningismus and peritonitis.

J Neurosurg 2001; 94: 202.

CSF Shunt Infections – Presenting Features in Children

Feature	V-P shunt[1]	V-A shunt[1]	Most common organisms	
Fever	95%	100%	Staph epidermidis SE	32-57%
Shunt malfunction	57%	14%	Staph. aureus SA	4-38%
Abdominal pain	48%	0	SA + Strep. viridans	4-15%
Meningismus	29%	0	Gram negatives ± SE	15% (3%)
Headache	14%	14%	SE + Enterococcus	7%
Irritability	19%	43%	SE + strep. pyogenes	4%
Nephritis	0	14%	Enterococcus/Candida	4%

[1] V-A – ventriculoatrial, V-P – ventriculoperitoneal

Infection 1993;21:89; *Pediatr Neurosurg* 1999;30:253.

Management of Shunt Malfunction/Infection

- Apply cardiac telemetry & pulse oximeter (risk of apnea, bradycardia)
- Head to toe examination with emphasis on shunt tract and neurologic exam.
- AP/Lateral films of skull, torso where shunt located, CT scan of the head (up to 24% will have CT read as unchanged/normal/smaller ventricles or negative)
- Shunt tap for pressure assessment, cell count, culture (do not perform LP in ED due to risk of herniation & ↑ rate of missed infection)
- Shunt failure requires surgery. Treat impending herniation as needed. Infection usually requires external ventricular drainage (60-68%) or externalization of shunt (25-33%), & empiric antibiotics until culture results return (vancomycin 15 mg/kg IV q6h **OR** nafcillin 150-200 mg/kg/d divided q4-6h) + (aminoglycoside **OR** rifampin) See page 83 for dosing recommendations.

Weakness

Upper motor neuron (UMN) lesions cause damage to the cortex (e.g., stroke), brain stem, or spinal cord. Lower motor neuron (LMN) lesions damage the anterior horn cells (e.g., poliomyelitis), the neuromuscular junction (e.g., myasthenia gravis, botulism toxin) or muscle (e.g., muscular dystrophies).

	Category	UMN disease	LMN disease
Differentiation of	Muscular deficit	Muscle groups	Individual muscles
upper motor neuron	Reflexes	Increased	Decreased/absent
from lower motor	Tone	Increased	Decreased
neuron disease	Fasciculations	Absent	Present
	Atrophy	Absent/minimal	Present

Ataxia

Ataxia is the incoordination of movement with normal strength. Disorders of the cerebellar hemispheres cause ipsilateral limb ataxia, while disorders of the vermis cause truncal ataxia. Other causes of acute ataxia include cerebral cortex disorders (frontal ataxia), peripheral sensory nerve and spinal cord disorders (sensory ataxia), labyrinth disorders (vestibular ataxia), metabolic, and toxin-induced ataxia.

Specific diseases causing ataxia

- Acute cerebellar ataxia - the most common cause of acute ataxia in children. This is a post-viral autoimmune ataxia typically occurring in 1-3 year olds 2-3 weeks after varicella, influenza, or coxsackie infections. This disorder causes a sudden onset of ataxia, paroxysmal vertigo, nystagmus in 50%, elevated CSF protein, mild CSF pleocytosis, and frequently dysarthria. Ataxia may persist for weeks to years in up to 1/3 of patients.

- Drug ingestion - Common drugs causing ataxia include phenytoin (and most anticonvulsants), alcohol, tricyclic antidepressants, sedatives, heavy metals (e.g., lead), insecticides and drugs of abuse (e.g., PCP).

- Neuroblastomas - Occult neuroblastomas can cause classic triad of symptoms with acute ataxia, opsoclonus (jerky, random eye movements), and myoclonus.

- Posterior fossa tumors - Direct cerebellar involvement or hydrocephalus

- Diseases causing weakness easily mistaken for ataxia including Guillain-Barre, transverse myelitis, tick paralysis, and myasthenia gravis.

- Other causes include head trauma, stroke, vasculitis, and congenital disorders.

Nutrition

Water comprises 75% of body weight in infants and 60% in adults.

Energy requirements A child < 12 months of age requires 105-115 kcal/kg/day. Breast milk or commercially prepared formulas are usually the sole source of energy and nutrients in the first few months of life. Semisolid foods (e.g., cereals) are usually introduced into the diet at 4-6 months of age and soft table foods at 1 year.

Breast milk Breast milk is preferred over formula by the American Academy of Pediatrics. Breast-fed infants have less mortality, respiratory infections, otitis media, and diarrhea compared with formula-fed infants. Breast-fed infants require fewer calories than formula-fed infants. Lactose is predominant carbohydrate in breast milk, although glucose and galactose are also found. Human milk has lower protein concentrations than cow's milk (0.9% vs. 3.4%), is more easily digested than cow milk as the casein:whey ratio is lower (40/60 vs. 80/20). A disadvantage of breast feeding is infant jaundice due to inhibitory effects of a progesterone on bilirubin conjugation. This physiologic jaundice generally appears after the third day of life, peaks in 1st week, and usually is associated with bilirubin levels of 10-27 mg/dl (although levels >15 may be concerning, see page 59). Maternal contraindications to breast feeding include maternal (1) eclampsia, (2) severe infection, (3) TB, (4) severe heart disease, (5) thyrotoxicosis, (6) diabetes mellitus, (6) chronic renal disease, or (7) severe puerperal depression. Mastitis is not a contraindication.

Infant formulas Most infant formulas supply 20 calories per ounce. The AAP recommends formulas with caloric distribution of 30-54% fat, 7-18% protein, and remainder from carbohydrates. If fluoridated drinking water not available, fluoride supplementation is recommended for all infants. Iron supplementation is recommended by AAP after 4 months due to normally depleted iron stores. Most formulas contain 1 mg/L iron & fortified formulas contain 10-12 mg/L.

Protein	Formulas
Bovine (cow) Normal GI tract	Enfamil (demineralized whey), Enfamil AR (has whey + thick formula), Follow-up (use > 4 mo), Lactofree[4], Similac, Similac PM 60:40 (low Ca/P required), Similac lactose free[4], Similac Neosure & Similac Special Care 20 or 24 (for premie - has whey)
Soy[1] Cow milk allergy	Alsoy[3], Follow-up Soy[4,5], Isomil[4,5], Isomil DF (short term use with diarrhea – has soy fiber), ProSobee[4,5], RCF[6]
Casein[1]	Alimentum[3], MJ3232A[6], Nutramigen, Portagen[3], Pregestimil[3]
Whey	Good Start, Enfamil, Similac - Neosure/Special Care above
Free amino acid[1]	Neocate (severe food allergies)

[1]food allergy, [2]fat malabsorption, [3]protein-fat malabsorption, [4]lactose malabsorption, [5]galactosemia, [6]severe carbohydrate (CHO) intolerance (CHO must be added)

Low birth weight infants
Preterm and low birth-weight infants require 120-180 kcal/kg/day and 3 g/kg/day of protein to maintain growth and adequate nutritional status. The composition of breast milk produced by preterm mothers is uniquely suited to preterm or low birth weight neonates, and differs substantially from that produced at term.

Weaning and mixed feeding Some begin at 5-6 months of age. During weaning, mothers can gradually replace one breast feeding at a time with a formula feed offered by bottle or cup. Weaning is more easily accepted by an infant who has already been spoon-fed some solid foods. By 12 months of age, most infants have settled into a schedule of 3-4 meals per day. While bovine milk formulas are acceptable, regular bovine milk should not be given until after 1 year of age. Caries can occur from repetitive, prolonged (e.g., overnight) sucking of bottles before 2 years of age.

First year feeding problems
Constipation is rare in breast-fed infants. Formulas high in fat and protein may promote constipation. For these infants, increasing amount of fluid or sugar by adding 1-2 teaspoons of _Karo_ syrup to 8 oz water is usually helpful. If > 4 months, add bulk such as cereal, vegetables, or fruit. Iron-fortified formula may be continued. _Colic_ is rare after 3 months of age.

Nutritional Disorders

Failure to thrive (FTT) Inadequate growth indicated by weight ≤ the 3rd-5th percentile on standard growth chart or < 80-85% of the median for that child's age or height. Risk factors: young mother (<17 y), social isolation, marital problems, and poverty.
Bovine milk allergy The prevalence of allergy to bovine (cow's) milk is 0.3% - 7.5%. Allergy is due to sensitivity to the primary protein in bovine milk, β-lactoglobulin. Infants with milk allergy usually present during the 1st 6 weeks of life with diarrhea, mucous or bloody stools, and occasional respiratory symptoms. Treatment is aimed at eliminating bovine milk protein from the diet and substituting soy-based (e.g., _Pregestimil_) or hydrolyzed casein formulas (e.g., _Nutramigen_). See formula discussion & choices page 105.

Normal Feeding Amount and Timing

Age	Volume of meal (ounces)	Frequency
0 - 2 weeks	2 - 3	q 2 - 3 hours
2 - 6 weeks	3 - 4	q 3 - 4 hours
1 - 3 months	5 - 6	q 4 - 5 hours
3 - 4 months	6 - 7	q 5 - 6 hours
4 - 8 months	7 - 8	q 6 - 7 hours
8 - 12 months	7 - 8	q 8 hours

Guidelines for Eye Exam and Vision Screening in Infants & Children

Age	Examination
0-2 years	• Examine eyelids/orbits/external anatomy • Assess pupils & red reflex. • <u>Alignment/Motility</u> and eye muscle balance. Above 3 months infants should begin to *fix on target* (e.g. toy) and follow it. *Corneal light reflex* should present symmetrically on both corneas in relation to anterior structures. If not muscle imbalance may present. • <u>Vision</u> – *Unilateral cover test*. At age where infant can fix on a target, cover one eye at a time as move toy around. Poor vision may cause child's objection to one eye in particular being covered.
3-5 years	• Perform above exam with vision and alignment tests below • Ophthalmoscopy may be possible after age 4 • <u>Alignment</u> – (1) *unilateral cover test* at 10 feet. First fix on distant object at 10 feet. Abnormal if 1 eye moves while other covered. Or (2) *random dot E stereo test* – place cards 40cm from child, place stereo glasses on child (over corrective glasses), randomly pace E card in front of one or other eye & have child point to card with raised E. **Abnormal** test if identifies E correctly < 4 of 6 attempts. • <u>Vision</u> - At 2 ½ to 3 years may vision test with nontested eye completely occluded using (1) tumbling E (point to direction of E), (2) HOTV test (match letters on wall chart to 8.5 X 11' testing board that also contains letters HOTV), (3) LH test or Allen card test (schematic objects). A testing distance of 10 feet is recommended for all tests. **Abnormal** if < 4 of 6 correct on 20 ft. line with either eye tested at 10 feet monocularly (i.e. < 10/20 or 20/40) **OR** 2 line difference between eyes even if passing range.
≥ 6 years	• Examination, ophthalmoscopy with vision, alignment tests below • <u>Alignment</u> – unilateral cover test or random dot E stereo test above. **Abnormal** - any eye movement with cover test **OR** < 4 of 6 correct with random dot E stereo test. • <u>Vision</u> - Snellen letters and numbers at 10 feet. **Abnormal** if < 4 of 6 correct on 15 foot line with either eye tested at 10 feet monocularly (i.e. < 10/15 or 20/30) **OR** if 2 line difference between eyes even if both are within passing range.

AAP. Pediatrics 1996; 98: 153.

Strabismus – Ocular Misalignment[1]

Esotropia – eye turned in or unable to abduct (e.g. lateral rectus/CN VI palsy)
Exotropia – eye turned out or unable to adduct (e.g. medial rectus/CN III palsy)
Hypotropia – eye turned down/upward gaze palsy (e.g. superior rectus/CN III palsy)
Hypertropia – eye turned up/downward gaze palsy (e.g. inferior rectus/CN III palsy or superior oblique palsy/CN IV)

[1] Emergency strabismus is more likely associated with double vision (if chronic, brain suppresses misaligned eye & no diplopia), & absence of complete and full eye movement.

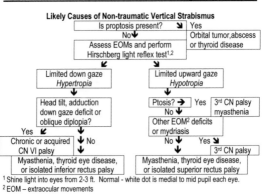

Likely Causes of Non-traumatic Vertical Strabismus

Is proptosis present? ↘	Yes
No ↓	Orbital tumor, abscess or thyroid disease
Assess EOMs and perform Hirschberg light reflex test[1,2]	

Limited down gaze
Hypertropia
↓
Head tilt, adduction down gaze deficit or oblique diplopia?
↙ Yes   ↓ No
Chronic or acquired CN VI palsy   ↓
Myasthenia, thyroid eye disease, or isolated inferior rectus palsy

Limited upward gaze
Hypotropia
↓
Ptosis? → Yes   3rd CN palsy myasthenia
No ↓
Other EOM[2] deficits or mydriasis
No ↓   Yes ↘
↓   3rd CN palsy
Myasthenia, thyroid eye disease, or isolated superior rectus palsy

[1] Shine light into eyes from 2-3 ft. Normal - white dot is medial to mid pupil each eye.
[2] EOM – extraocular movements

Likely Causes of Non-traumatic Horizontal Strabismus

Is proptosis present? ↘	Yes
No ↓	Orbital tumor, abscess or thyroid disease
Assess EOMs and perform Hirschberg light reflex test[1,2]	

Limited abduction
Esotropia
↓
CNS trauma, neuro deficit, ↑ICP, systemic illness, papilledema
Yes ↙   ↓ No
CN VI palsy   ↓
Myasthenia, thyroid eye disease

Limited adduction
Exotropia
↓
Ptosis? → Yes   3rd CN palsy myasthenia
No ↓
Other EOM[2] deficits or mydriasis
↓   Yes ↘
↓   3rd CN palsy myasthenia thyroid eye dz
No ↓
Medial rectus palsy, thyroid eye disease internuclear ophthalmoplegia (brainstem) myasthenia gravis

[1] Shine light into eyes from 2-3 ft. Normal - white dot is medial to mid pupil each eye.
[2] EOM – extraocular movements

Most Comm Etiology of Pediatric Cranial Nerve Palsy

	3rd nerve	4th nerve	6th nerve	Multiple Any Combination (3,4,6)
Trauma	40%	37%	42%	56%
Unknown	17%	21%	15%	-
Neoplasm	14%	5%	3%	17%
Opht. migraine	9%	-	-	-
Post surgical	9%	5%	1%	6%
Meningitis	3%	5%	2%	6%
Hydrocephalus	-	10%	2%	-
Aneurysm	-	-	-	11%
Viral infection	-	-	3%	-
Other[1]	9%	16%	14%	6%

[1]Other – thyroid/granulomatous/demyelinating dz, myasthenia, infection, Guillain Barre (Miller-Fisher variant)   *Am J Ophthalmol* 1992;114:568.

Unequal Pupils (Anisocoria) Evaluation[1,2]

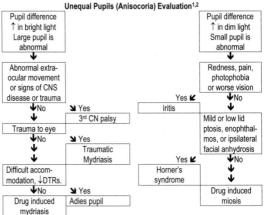

[1] See page 141 for drugs causing bilateral mydriasis or miosis.

[2] If no difference in pupils in light or dark, anisocoria may be physiologic.

Orthopedics - Arthritis & Joint Fluid & Infections

Analysis of Joint Fluid

	Noninflammatory	Inflammatory	Septic	Hemorrhagic
Clarity	Clear	Cloudy	Purulent/turbid	Bloody
Color	Yellow	Yellow	Yellow	Red/brown
WBC/ml	<200-2000	200-100,000	> 50,000	< 200[2]
PMN (%)	< 25%	> 75%	> 75%	< 25%
Glucose[1]	95-100%	80-100%	< 50%	100%
Culture	Negative	Negative	Pos. > 50%	Negative
Disease	DJD,trauma,rheumatic fever,osteochondritis	Crystal, spondyloarthopathy,Lyme, Reiters, TB, fungi, viral,RA[3]	Septic arthritis	Trauma, bleeding diathesis, neoplasm

[1] Joint/serum glucose X 100%, [2] Pure blood, joint = serum WBC, [3]Rheumatoid arthritis

Etiology of Arthritis Based on Number of Involved Joints[1]

Monoarthritis (1 joint)	Trauma, tumor, septic, gout or pseudogout	Lyme disease, avascular necrosis, osteoarthritis (acutely)
Oligoarthritis (2-3 joints)	Lyme, Reiter's rheumatic fever	Gonococcal, ankylosing spondylitis, gout (polyarticular)
Polyarthritis (> 3 joints)	Rheumatoid, lupus, viral (rubella, hepatitis),	Serum sickness, septic (neonate, immunocompromised)

[1] Migratory arthritis causes: gonococcal, viral, rheumatic fever, Lyme, lupus, subacute endocarditis, mycoplasma, histoplasmosis, coccidiomycosis, Henoch-Schonlein purpura, serum sickness (esp. cefaclor), sepsis (S. aureus, streptococcus, meningococcus)

Septic Arthritis

Overview – neonatal = Group B strep, S. aureus, gram neg. > 2 mo, S. aureus, Strep. gram neg., Neisseria, Salmonella (esp. sickle cell), Pseudomonas(puncture rubber). 90% - 1 joint (knee>hip>ankle), multiple if neonate. Pseudoparalysis & irritability occur in young, & pain/↓ ROM older. Joint usually held in position max. distention. ↑ resistance to movement. US - effusion in 85% septic hips. (also trans. synovitis). Joint culture+ in 50-80% *Management* – (1) IV antibiotics (see page 82), (2) repeat aspiration, (3) surgical drainage if (a) hip, (b) ↑ debris, fibrin, loculation in joint space or (c) no improvement within 3 days IV antibiotics

Presenting Features[1]	
• Mean age	4 years
• Age < 2 years	46-69%
• Median duration symptom	3 days
• Recent URI/trauma	53/31%
• Associated osteomyelitis	22%
• Temperature > 101F	~75%
• ↑Sedimentation rate (ESR)	60-90%
• Mean ESR	36-56
• ↑ C reactive protein	82-95%
• ↑ Serum WBC	46-60%
• Xray normal (except neonate – hip subluxation)	~80%
• Technetium scan positive	70-90%
• MRI + (better than US at telling septic jt. vs synovitis)	88%

[1] See page 121 for algorithm discriminating between septic vs transient synovitis of hip.
Ped EM Care 199940.*Sws Med Wk* 2001; 575.*Peds ID J* 1986;669;1992;88;1997;411.
AJDC 1987;898,*Ann E Med* 1992;1418.*Rad Clin N Am* 2001:267.*J Ped Ortho*1989;9:579.

Osteomyelitis (see page 112 for vertebral osteomyelitis)

Overview – In neonate, Gp B strep, S. aureus, gram neg. In neonate, most common features are pseudoparalysis (64%), tenderness (55%), fever (32%), red (32%), & irritability (36%). Infants may have paradoxic irritability (pain ↑ with holding) if older, S. aureus > strep > gram neg. Most common sites: femur > tibia > foot > humerus > pelvis. *Management* – (1) IV antibiotics (see page 80). (2) Surgery may be indicated for (a) abscess formation, (b) bacteremia beyond 72 h IV antibiotics, (c) sinus tract, or (d) sequestra presence.	Presenting Features (exclude neonate)	
	● Mean age (years)	5.9
	● Age < 5 years	50%
	● Complaint of pain/swelling	65/54%
	● Local tender/warmth/red	1/3 each
	● Fever by Hx or exam	75-85%
	● ↑sedimentation rate (ESR)	89-92%
	● Mean ESR	42-61
	● ↑ C reactive protein	98%
	● ↑ serum WBC	31-43%
	● Normal WBC and ESR	< 5%
	● Xray normal (esp. 1st 10 d)	42%
	● Technetium scan abnl	82-95%
	● MRI abnormal	88-100%

*AJDC*1991;65,*Peds*1994;59.*Ped IDJ* 1987;29.1990; 416, 1992;88. *Rad Clin NA* 12001;251 *J Pediatr Orthop* 1990; 10: 649.

Back Pain

	Etiology	< 12 years	≥ 12 years
Etiology of Back Pain in 225 Children Presenting to a Pediatric ED	Musculoskeletal (trauma, strain)	57%	43%
	Infection(viral,pneumonia,UTI [5%])[1]	13%	17%
	Idiopathic	12%	13%
	Sickle cell disease	14%	13%
	Psychogenic	2%	2%
	Other (gallstones, pancreas, renal)	2%	13%

[1]If fever, 36% had source (meningitis, lung, pharyngitis, PID, UTI), 32% virus, 18% sickle crisis. See below + pg 112 for discitis, vert. osteo, epidural abscess.*Clin Pediatr* 1999; 401.

Discitis

Overview – intervertebral disc infection due to hematogenous spread to vascular channels in cartilage of intervertebral disc space that disappear later in life. 1/3 of patients have + cultures (blood or disc) for S. aureus. Most are culture negative. Xrays are abnormal in 76%[1]. MRI is diagnostic procedure of choice. *Management* – (1) exclude more serious disease (osteomyelitis, abscess, tumor or other peritoneal, retroperitoneal abscess). (2) antibiotic use debatable; if used, initiate with nafcillin or *Ancef*.	Presenting Features	
	● Age ≤ 2.5 years	75%
	● Refuse/difficult walking	56%
	● Back/neck pain (100% >3y)	25-42%
	● Abdominal pain	3-22%
	● Ave symptom duration (d)	5-22
	● Hx fever or T > 100.3°F	28-47%
	● Tender back	50%
	● Lumbosacral involvement	78-82%
	● Serum WBC > 10,500	50%
	● Mean ESR (mm/hour)	39-42
	● Abnormal bone scan	72-90%
	● Abnormal MRI[2]	90-100%

[1]↓ disc space, eroded vert end plates, [2]Negative MRIs occurred 1 month after admit.
Pediatrics 2000; 105: 1299.; *Clin Orthop* 1991; 266: 70.

Epidural Abscess (Spinal)

Overview – Abscess in spinal epidural space usually involves posterior aspect of epidural space (86%), esp. lumbar region extending to 7 vertebral levels. S. aureus is cause in 79%, strep. in 8%, followed by gram negatives/mixed flora. Occasionally, *Mycobacterium tuberculosis* is cause. Source is hematogenous in ½ - seeded by skin or soft tissue site. ¼ had spine trauma precipitant. *Management* – (1) IV antibiotics (nafcillin + a 3rd generation cephalosporin until cultures return) X 2 weeks (6-8 weeks if coexisting osteomyelitis) – if methicillin resistance add vancomycin. (2) surgical drainage.	Presenting Features	
	● Mean age	8 years
	● Mean symptom duration	8-9 days
	● Limb weakness	78%
	● Fever	63%
	● Back pain	54%
	● Complete paralysis	45%
	● Partial paralysis	33%
	● Sphincter disturbance	38%
	● Spine tenderness	27%
	● Sensory level	24%
	● Abnormal plain films[1]	14-50%%
	● Cerebrospinal fluid WBC count elevated	37%
	● Elevated serum WBC	85%
	● Abnormal myelogram	100%
	● Abnormal MRI	92-100%

[1] Most commonly - loss of intervertebral disc height

Neurology 1980;30:844. *Clin Infect Dis*2001;32:9.;*Pediatr Infect Dis J*1993;12:1007.

Vertebral Osteomyelitis

Etiology – S. aureus > S. epidermidis, gram negatives, Bartonella. Infection occurs when organisms settle in low flow vasculature near subchondral plate. Patients are generally older and more ill-appearing than those with discitis. Recent trauma is noted in 14%. *Management* – Diagnose by MRI, although technetium scanning may be more useful in very young with non-localized pain. IV antibiotics (see osteomyelitis). Surgery may be indicated for (a) abscess formation, (b) bacteremia or systemic illness beyond 48-72 h IV antibiotics, (c) sinus tract, (d) sequestra presence, (e) progressive neurologic deficit, (f) progressive vertebral body collapse or kyphosis.	Presenting Features	
	● Median age (years)	6-8
	● Age ≤ 2.5 years	14%
	● Ave symptom duration (d)	33
	● History fever	54-79%
	● Back/neck pain (all ages)	64%
	● Prior infection (lung, skin)	29%
	● Back trauma	21%
	● Limp	14%
	● Abdominal, shoulder, rib pain or incontinence	7% each
	● Hip or flank pain	8%
	● Temperature > 102	79%
	● Paraspinal mass	11%
	● Mean WBC (cells/mm³)	12,600
	● WBC > 11,000 (cells/mm³)	64%
	● Mean ESR (mm/hour)	46
	● Abnormal Xray[1]	46%
	● Abnormal bone scan	85-95%
	● Abnormal MRI	96-100%

Pediatrics 2000; 105: 1129; *Pediatr Infect Dis J* 1993; 12: 228.

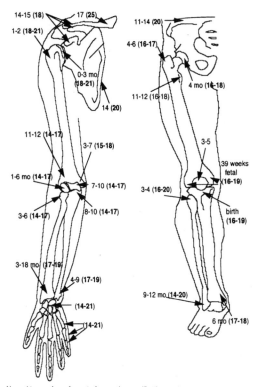

14-15 (18) 17 (25)
1-2 (18-21)
0-3 mo (18-21)
14 (20)
11-12 (14-17)
3-7 (15-18)
1-6 mo (14-17)
7-10 (14-17)
3-6 (14-17)
8-10 (14-17)
3-18 mo (17-19)
4-9 (17-19)
(14-21)
(14-21)

11-14 (20)
4-6 (16-17)
4 mo (16-18)
11-12 (16-18)
3-5
39 weeks fetal (16-19)
3-4 (16-20)
birth (16-19)
9-12 mo (14-20)
6 mo (17-18)

Normal type – Age of onset of secondary ossification centers.
(Bold type in parenthesis) – Age of physeal closure.
All ages are in years unless otherwise specified.

Extremity Injuries

Salter-Harris/Ogden-Harris Physeal Fracture Classification

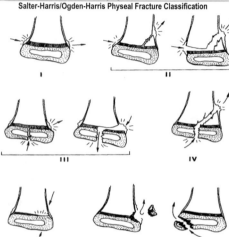

With permission Strange GR. *Pediatric Emergency Medicine*. A comprehensive study guide. McGraw Hill1996.

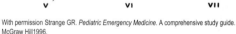

Salter I	Complete separation of the epiphysis and most of physis from metaphysis due to shearing force. Usually no long term growth problems (except distal/proximal femur, proximal radius, and proximal tibia - can prematurely close with growth arrest)
Salter II	Fracture line extends along physis into metaphysis. Usually > 10 yr. Generally have good prognosis.
Salter III	Fracture line extends physis through epiphysis to articular surface.
Salter IV	Fracture at articular surface crosses epiphysis to metaphysis. Most III and IV injuries will require exact reduction and orthopedic consult.
Salter V	Longitudinal compression of growth plate
Ogden VI	Peripheral shear to borders of growth plate
Ogden VII	Intraarticular epiphyseal injury, ligament pulling off distal epiphysis
Ogden VIII	Fracture through metaphysis with circulation disruption
Ogden IX	Fracture with loss of periosteum

Upper Extremity Injuries

Management (If Closed, No Neurovascular injury, No Rotational Deformity)

Shoulder Clavicle

Scapula fracture (fx)	• 75% have other serious injuries with mortality up to 14% • Surgery if body fx displaced > 10 mm, neck + clavicle fx, displaced coracoid fx + distal clavicle or AC joint injury, acromial fx + subacromial narrowing, glenoid neck fx + > 10 mm displaced or ≥ 40°, glenoid rim + shoulder sublux/instability, or glenoid fossa displaced > 3-5 mm
Clavicle fracture (fx)	• Middle 3rd – Nonoperative, sling or figure of eight. Medial 3rd – Usually a Salter Harris I or II injury and mimics a sterno-clavicular dislocation. If post displacement, exclude mediastinal injury. Reduce under general anesthesia. Distal 3rd –Immobilize nondisplaced as per middle 3rd. Grossly displaced (types IV-VI) require surgery (esp. > 13 yo)

Humerus/Elbow

Proximal fracture (fx) (80% of humerus growth occurs here)	• Proximal humeral ossification cannot be seen on Xray until 6 months, greater tuberosity at 1-3 years, lesser tuberosity by 4-5 years. • Salter I - mostly < 5 years, with Salter II occurring in older. III/IV rare. • Majority of severely displaced fractures should be treated by sling and swathe immobilization. Acceptable alignment for closed management (if patient has open physis or is within 1-2 years of physeal closure) is (1) complete displacement, (2) ≤ 3cm of overriding, and (3) ≤ 60 degrees of angulation. Surgery if (1) open fracture, tenting of skin, displacement greater than (1-3) above, or neurovascular injury.
Little League Shoulder	• Osteochondrosis/traction apophysitis proximal humerus. Overuse from throwing. Xray - normal or wide physis. Generally treat with rest.
Humeral shaft fracture	• Radial nerve injury most common with distal/mid 3rd. 78-100% recovery • ≤ 3 years old, accept 45 degrees of angulation. Treat with sling & swathe or Velpau bandage. • > 3 years old, accept complete displacement & 2 cm shortening. If prox shaft, 25-30° of angulation is acceptable. If mid shaft, 20° of angulation is acceptable. If distal 1/3 shaft, 15-20°degrees of angulation is acceptable. Treat with coaptation splint/sling or hanging arm cast.
Supracondylar Fracture *Gartland Classification & also denote if extension (95% of cases) - or flexion injury*	• Splint undiagnosed/unreduced in 30° of flexion. Posterior-laterally displaced fracture may injure radial nerve. Medially displaced fracture (more common) may injure brachial artery & median nerve. • <u>Type I</u> – nondisplaced + normal Baumann angle (angle physeal line lat. condyle/humeral shaft = 75-80°). -IA or [1B if commination, collapse, min angle] long arm post splint, elbow > 90°, forearm neutral or pronate • <u>Type II</u> – displaced, intact posterior cortex. Treatment: closed reduction with pin fixation for most • <u>Type III</u> – completely displaced or no cortical contact. 10-20% have absent pulse. Treatment: pinning/surgery

Transphyseal	• Closed reduction and pin fixation required for most
Lateral condyle fracture	• Milch (I) extends to capitellum ossification center, (II) medial to trochlea • Stages - articular surface (I) intact, (II) disrupted, (III) displaced/rotated • Nondisplaced – long arm splint, elbow 90°, supinate or neutral forearm • Displaced ≥ 2 to 4 mm – reduction & surgery
Medial epicondyle (Med. epic.)	• Ulnar nerve injury rate is 10-16%. If associated elbow dislocation, up to 50% may have an ulnar nerve injury. • Displaced < 5 mm – post. splint, long arm cast or sling • Displaced ≥ 5 mm, intraarticular fragment, incarcerated fragment, ulnar nerve injury, or late instability may require surgery
Med. epic. apophysitis	• Little league elbow: pain/tender medial elbow from repeat valgus stress. Generally, treat with rest. Although, displacement may need surgery.

Radius(R)/Ulna/Carpal/Metacarpal/Phalangeal

Radial head subluxation (nursemaid's elbow)	• Injury in 6 months to 5 year old due to annular ligament slipping over radial head margin becoming caught between radial head & capitellum. • Treat by (1) flex elbow 90° & supinate forearm or (2) hyperpronate wrist/forearm followed by elbow flexion
Olecranon fracture	• Nondisplaced – post splint elbow in partial extension ≤ 75-80° • Displaced – > 3 mm + extraarticular, closed reduction/immobilization. If displaced > 3 mm + intraarticular or if comminuted requires surgery.
Radial head fractures	• Ossification of radial head epiphysis begins at 5 years. The radial head is largely cartilaginous and rarely injured.
Radial neck fractures	• 50% of radial neck fractures have other associated fractures or injury. Most are Salter Harris I and II injuries. • If < 10 years old, accept ≤ 45 degrees of angulation, and < 33% displacement (translation). If ≥ 10 years old, accept ≤ 30 degrees of angulation & ≤ 3mm displacement (translation) • If do not meet above criteria, closed or open reduction may be required.
Radioulnar (both bones) fracture	• ± Entrapped median, anterior interosseus (FPL, lateral FDPs, pronator quadratus), superficial radial nerve (sensory dorsal, thumb web space) • Plastic deformation (bowing fractures). Treat by reducing plastic deformation under general anesthesia. • Greenstick fracture (Complete disruption of only one cortex with plastic deformation of the other cortex. Rotation & angular deformity present.) Treat by closed reduction by reversing the deforming forces (after appropriate anesthesia. If apex volar (distal fragment dorsally angulated), pronate forearm and apply volar surface pressure to fracture apex. If apex dorsal (distal fragment is volarly angulated), supinate forearm and apply dorsal surface pressure to fracture apex. Apply sugar tong or bivalved long arm cast. • Complete shaft fracture – Treat by closed reduction. If ≤ 8 yo, ≤ 15°of prox/midshaft angulation is acceptable, if > 8 years old, ≤ 10° of mid & prox. shaft angulation. At any age, < 20-30° malrotation is acceptable.

Monteggia fracture *Bado classification*	• 25% have post. interosseous nerve injury (wrist extensors – not ECRL) • <u>Type I</u> – anterior dislocation radial head, fracture ulnar diaphysis. • <u>Type II</u> – (associated with ulnar nerve injury) - post. dislocation radial head, ulnar diaphyseal or metaphyseal fracture + posterior angulation. • <u>Type III</u> – lat. or anterolat. dislocation radial head, ulnar metaphyseal fx. • <u>Type IV</u> – anterior dislocation of radial head with ulnar/radial fracture at same levels or with radial fracture distal to ulnar fracture. • Manage primarily based on ulnar fracture. If ulna plastic deformation or incomplete ulnar fracture (greenstick/buckle), closed reduction with up to 10° angle acceptable followed by radial head reduction. Pinning or surgery may be needed if complete transverse, oblique or comminuted fracture of ulna or unable to reduce radial head.
Distal radius fracture	• <u>Physeal</u> – If nondisplaced, immobilization. If displaced or neuro-vascular compromise, closed reduction and pinning. Open reduction if irreducible, open, displaced Salter Harris III/IV fracture, compartment syndrome or acute carpal tunnel syndrome. • <u>Metaphyseal</u> – if nondisplaced, torus/buckle immobilize. Reduction to following goals is required if displaced fracture. If age 4-9, sagittal angulation 20° male, 15° female, frontal 15° (both) If age 9-11, sagittal angulation 15° male, 10° female, frontal 5° (both) If age 11-13, sagittal angulation 10° male, 10° female, frontal 0° (both) If age >13, sagittal angulation 5° male, 0° female, frontal 0° (both) Immobilize with sugar tong cast Open reduction is reserved for fractures that are irreducible or open.
Galeazzi fractures	• Fracture distal radius with distal radioulnar disruption. <u>Type I</u> – dorsal displacement distal radius <u>Type II</u> – volar displacement of distal radius • Treat: closed reduction and above elbow cast in full supination
Scaphoid	• Immobilize long arm thumb spica if nondisplaced. If displaced,ORIF
Metacarpal fractures	• (1) <u>Epiphyseal/Physeal</u> – many are irreducible or unstable requiring pin or surgery; (2) <u>Neck</u> – most can be reduced and splinted in "safe position" – maximum MCP flexion with extension of IP joints placing collateral ligaments at max length & preventing contracture (3) <u>Shaft</u> – closed reduction for most with MCP 70°, wrist extended 10-15°, PIP free (4) <u>Base</u> – many are high energy with ↑ tissue disruption. Fx/dislocations usually require surgery.
Thumb metacarpal fractures	• Head/Shaft –closed reduction unless intraarticular or complex shaft • Base – <u>Type A</u> (metaphyseal) <u>Type B</u> (Salter II with metaphyseal piece on medial side and lateral angulation of shaft), <u>Type C</u> (Salter II with metaphyseal piece on lateral side with medial angulation of shaft), <u>Type D</u> (Salter III – pediatric Bennett's) • Type A/ B usually can be treated with closed reduction. Many Type C and most (± all) Type D + Salter IV fx require open reduction.

Extremity Injuries – Pelvis & Lower Extremity

Classification of Pediatric Pelvic Fractures[1]

Torode and Zieg Classification[a]		Tile and Pennal Classification	
Type I	Avulsion fractures (fx)	Type A	Stable fractures
Type II	Iliac wing fracture	A1	Avulsion fractures
IIa	Separated iliac apophysis	A2	Undisplaced wing/ring fx
IIb	Fracture bony iliac wing	A3	Transverse fracture of
Type III	Simple ring fractures		sacrum or coccyx
IIIa	Pubis fx,disrupted symphysis posterior structures stable	Type B	Partially unstable fx
		B1	Open book fx
IIIb	Acetabular fx, no ring fx	B2	Lat. compress (triradiate)
Type IV	Fx with unstable segment ring disruption fracture	B3	Bilateral type B injuries
		Type C	Unstable pelvic ring
IVa	Bilateral sup/inferior rami	C1	Unilateral fractures
IVb	Anterior rami or symphysis + posterior fx (e.g. sacrum)	C1-1	Ilium fracture
		C1-2	Dislocation ± fx SI joint
		C1-3	Sacral fracture
IVc	Fx - unstable piece between ant. ring pelvis/acetabulum	C2	Bilat fx (1 type B/1 typeC)
[a]Class does not include acetabular fx.		C3	Bilateral type C fractures

Torode class	Mortality	GU injury	Other Fx[2]	Neuro. injury	Abd surgery
II	0%	6%	39%	61%	11%
III	3%	26%	49%	57%	13%
IV	13%	38%	56%	56%	40%

[1] Once triradiate cartilage closed, adult classification (Tile) and treatment is used.
[2] Fx- Other fractures (non-pelvic)   *J Pediatr Orthop* 1985; 5: 76. & 2002; 22: 22.

Avulsion Fractures of Pelvis/Proximal Femur

Location (relative frequency)	Mechanism
Ischial tuberosity (38-54%)	forceful hamstring contraction - jumping
Ant sup. iliac spine (19-32%)	forceful sartorius contraction – kicking/sprint
Ant inf. iliac spine (18-22%)	forceful rectus femoris contraction - kicking
Lesser trochanter (9%)	forceful psoas contract – sprint, jump, kick, skating
Iliac crest (1-3%)	contract abdomen/obliques– kicking twisting rotate
Symphysis pubis (0-3%)	contraction leg adductors - swim, kick, jump, run

Management –Rest, no weight bear for ≥ 3-7 d, then gradual weight with crutches, then limited exercise for 2-4 weeks. Surgery if displaced > 2 cm, chronic pain + excess callus (esp. ischial), Rockwood <u>Fractures in Child</u> 2001;<u>Skel Rad</u> 2001;127.*Rad Clin N Am* 1997;747.

High Yield Criteria for Knee, Ankle, & Pelvic Radiographs in the ED

Pelvic crit.	Painful or tender/abraded/contused pelvis, GCS < 15 or distracting injury
Knee criteria	(1) Unable to flex 90° or (2) unable to bear weight in the ED
Ankle criteria	(1) Unable to bear weight immediately after injury or (2) unable to take 4 steps in the ED or (3) tender along inferior or posterior edge of malleolus

Knee criteria were 92-100% sensitive (*Ped Emerg Care* 1998;185&2001;401) ankle criteria were 100% sensitive (*Arch Ped Adoles Med* 1995; 149: 255. & *Acad EM* 1999; 6:1005) & pelvic criteria were 99-100% sensitive. *Pediatr Emerg Care* 2001; 17: 15.

Acetabulum/Femur	
Acetabulum	• <u>Type I</u> – small fragments ± hip dislocate; (II) – linear fx ± pelvic fx not displaced; (III) – linear fx, hip unstable; (IV) – central fx dislocation. • Nondisplaced/minimally displaced/stable (≤ 1 mm) – bed rest, non-weight bearing. Traction or surgery if unstable or displaced > 1 mm
Hip fracture *Delbet classification*	• <u>Type I</u> – transepiphyseal ± acetabular dislocation, <u>type II</u> – transcervical (femoral neck), <u>type III</u> – cervicotrochanteric (base femoral neck), <u>type IV</u> – intertrochanteric. Management consists of reduction if needed, and spica cast or surgery depending on patient age & specific injury.
Femur shaft	• Classify based on location (prox, mid, distal 3ʳᵈ), configuration (spiral, oblique, transverse), angle, degree of communication, shortening (unacceptable if > 3 cm), open or closed. • Depending on injury & age, Pavlik harness, spica, traction, surgery.
Distal femur	• Peroneal nerve & rare popliteal artery injury. 23-38% have ligament injuries (usually anterior cruciate). Classify via (1) Salter Harris (60% type II), (2) displacement (med, lat, ant, post [↑ popliteal artery injury]), & (3) age (infant & juvenile [↑ risk growth disturbance], adolescent. • If nondisplaced, long leg cast with knee in 15-20° with molding forces opposite to injury mechanism & intact periosteal hinge tightened. • If distal femoral metaphyseal/physeal fx – closed reduction (general anesthesia) in sagittal plane to < 20° if < 10 years and less if > 10 y. Varus/valgus alignment should be < 5° with no rotation. Irreducible type II & most displaced type III, IV, & V fractures require open reduction.

Knee	
Patella & patellar sleeve	• <u>Patella</u> - If nondisplaced, intact retinaculum, external immobilization + long leg cast in near extension. Surgery indicated if > 4 mm articular displacement, articular step off > 3 mm or comminution. • <u>Sleeve fx</u> - avulsion distal pole patella with sleeve or articular cartilage, periosteum, & retinaculum (esp. 8-12 years old). Often missed on Xray. Need MRI to diagnose. Treat surgically.
Tibial tuberosity *Ogden classification*	• <u>Type I</u> – distal to junction of ossification of prox tibia & tuberosity, <u>Type II</u> – junction of ossification of prox tibia & tuberosity, <u>Type III</u> – extend to joint, assoc. with displaced ant. fragment & discontinuation joint surface • Surgery is indicated for all except type I with minimal displacement.
Tibial spine *Meyers-McKeever classification*	• <u>Type I</u> – min. displaced, slight ant. margin elevation, <u>Type II</u> – anterior 3ʳᵈ to ½ of avulsed fragment elevated, <u>Type III</u> – avulsed fragment completely elevated with no bony apposition remaining. • Type 1 – long leg cast, knee 10-20° (if tense hemarthrosis, ± needle aspiration), Type II – closed reduction, Type III – open reduction
Osgood Schlatter	• Tibial tubercle apophysitis – traction apophysitis of ant. tibial tubercle, in early puberty. Treat with rest, hamstring stretch & quad strengthening.
Jumper's knee	• Sinding-Larson-Johansson = apophysitis inferior pole patella. Pain if run, jump. Treat - rest, patellar tendon straps may be tried.
Osteochondritis dissecans of femur	• Medial epicondyle of femur. Occurs in males > females aged 12-16. Osteochondral bone separates from healthy bone. Progressive, joint pain. Immobilize most, surgery if loose body, or not better after 6 mo.

	Tibia/Fibula/Ankle/Foot
Proximal tibial physis	• Popliteal artery injury in 3-7%. Compartment syndrome also occurs • Classify using Salter Harris. Nonoperative if non or minimally displaced. Most others require surgery. If reduction, general anesthesia.
Tibia & fibula shaft fracture	• Associated - compartment syndrome of lower extremity. Proximal metaphyseal/distal tibia fractures can cause anterior tibial artery injury. • Prox tibia fx – if nondisplaced, long leg splint/cast with knee nearly full extension + varus mold. If displaced, admit + closed reduction in OR. • Diaphyseal – displaced, closed reduction. Surgery –unstable, shortening uncorrected by closed treatment, displaced fx in skeletally mature.
Toddler fracture	• History minor trauma, in child < 5 years old (mean age 27 months). Undisplaced oblique/spiral distal tibia fx, may require oblique Xray to ID. • Immobilize in bent knee 30-40°, long leg cast.
Distal tibia & fibula fractures	• Group I: Low risk injuries including avulsion fractures, and minor epiphyseal separations (e.g. Salter Harris I and II). Usually managed by closed reduction and casting. • Group II: High risk injuries including fractures through the epiphyseal plate (Salter Harris III, IV, and V), and transitional fractures (occur during time of physeal closure – adolescence). Examples of transitional fx: (1) *Juvenile Tillaux* [Salter III lateral tibia fx due to external foot rotation] and (2) triplanar [appears as Juvenile Tillaux seen on AP Xray + Salter II fx distal tibia primarily seen on lateral Xray]. Group II injuries are usually intraarticular with joint instability. Treat most Group II injuries by open reduction internal fixation to achieve accurate anatomic reduction.
Talus fracture	• Neck fx most common. Nondisplaced - long leg cast knee flexed so no weight bearing. Surgery if ≥ 3 mm dorsal displace or ≥ 5° varus rotation.
Calcaneus fx	• Immobilize most without reduction of weight bearing. If severe displacement/intraarticular ± surgery (not needed as often as in adults)
Sever's disease	• Calcaneal apophysitis. Pain at Achilles insertion. Chronic heel pain. Treat - 1 cm heel pad, stretching, resolves as apophysis fuses ~ 12 y.
Kohler's disease	• Avascular necrosis of tarsal navicular from repeated trauma to maturing epiphysis. Most common at 4-7 y. Treat with rest or immobilization.
Metatarsal fracture	• Compartment syndrome can occur if marked trauma/swelling. • Shaft/Neck – Immobilize in short leg walking cast. Wire fixation/surgery may be required if unstable (esp. 1st and 5th MT). 5th MT base – (1) avulsion fx of tuberosity - extraarticular requiring immobilization/NSAIDs (2) prox metaphyseal-diaphyseal (Jones) fx. – nondisplaced immobilize – Ortho follow up, if displaced ± surgery (3) diaphyseal stress fx.
Freiberg's infarction	• Osteochondrosis of 2nd MT head. 75% female esp. > 13. MT pad, short leg cast. Surgery if persistent pain, MT deformed or MT ↓ ROM.

Hip Pain & Limping

Differential of Painful Hip

Features	Toxic synovitis	Legg-Calve Perthes	Septic arthritis	Slipped capital femoral epiphysis
Age (y)	1½ -12	4-9	< 2, but any age	8-16
Sex (M:F)	3:2	5:1	1:1	2:1
History	prior URI	minimally painful	fever, ± prior URI	obesity in 88%
Physical exam	↓ hip abduction & rotation	limited hip abduction	hip often held flexed, abducted	Trendelenberg gait, hip ER with flexion
X-rays	enlarged medial joint space	subchondral lucency femur	↑ joint space, fem head lat subluxed	line fem. neck crosses <10% epiphysis
Ultrasound	effusion ~90%	no effusion	effusion	no effusion
WBC/ESR	normal	normal	elevated	normal

Differentiating Septic Arthritis From Transient Synovitis of Hip	Clinical Feature	Probability of Septic Arthritis	
	• History fever > 101.3 (38.5C)	No listed features	0.2%
	• No weight bearing	Any one feature	3%
	• ESR ≥ 40 mm/h[1]	Any two features	40%
	• Serum WBC > 12,000 cells/mm³	Any three features	93.1%
		All four features	99.6%

[1] Sedimentation rate   *J Bone Joint Surg A* 1999; 81: 1662.

Etiology of Limp in Children < 14 years Old Presenting to a Pediatric ED

Location of pain		Final Diagnoses			
Hip	34%	Toxic synovitis	40%	Cellulitis/adenitis	2%
No pain	21%	Unknown	29%	Toddler's fracture	1%
Knee	19%	Strain/overuse	18%	Other fx, Kohlers	2%
Leg-not hip/knee	18%	Reactive arthritis/HSP	3%	Malignancy	1%
Not localized	7%	Legg-Calve-Perthes	2%	SCFE	<1%
Back	2%	Osteomyelitis	2%	Osgood Schlatter	<1%

[1]Prospective, no recent trauma, [2] ST - soft tissue   *J Bone Joint Surg Br* 1999; 81: 102.

Limp Classification & Associated Etiology

Antalgic gait	↓ Stance phase due to pain to weight bearing extremity	Fx, septic arthritis, synovitis, osteo. dessicans
Prox muscle weakness	↑ Lordosis, Gower's sign–child must climb up by pushing off with hands w low ext.	Muscular dystrophy
Spastic gait	Spastic hamstrings restrict knee ext. Gait scissoring (excess hip abduct) - running	Cerebral palsy (CP)
Steppage gait	Foot drop - exaggerated hip, knee flexion during swing phase to clear dropped foot	Neuro disease or deficit with ↓ankle dorsiflexion
Stooped gait	Walk with bilateral ↑ hip flexion	PID,appendicitis, abscess
Toe walking	Walks on toes	CP, heel fx or FB, Sever's
Trendelenberg gait	Downward pelvic tilt during swing phase due to weakness/spasm contralat. gluteus	LC Perthes, SCFE, congenital hip dislocation
Vaulting gait	Knee hyperextends/locks at end of stance phase, child vaults over extremity	Illness with weak quadriceps femoris

Tumors (Bony & Cartilagenous Malignancy/Non-malignancy)

	Malignant (each may ↑ESR/alkaline phosphatase)
Ewing's sarcoma	• *Features* – age 10-20. Usually axial/pelvis or lower extremity. 50% have symptoms for 6 mo pre-diagnosis. 61% palpable mass. • *Xray* – mottled, periosteal new bone formation – "onion peeling"
Histiocytosis X *Benign or life-threatening*	• *Features* – age 5-10. 80% solitary, 6% multiple granulomas, 9% Hand-Schuller-Christian dz. Skull > femur. Skin (seborrheic dermatitis), gums, exophthalmos, lung, immune disease can occur. • *Xray* – punched out, moth eaten lesions ± periosteal elevation.
Leukemia & Metastasis	• Leukemia → metaphysis radiolucency 8-80%, osteopenia 16-41%, lytic lesions 11-39%. Wilms, neuroblastoma esp occur < 5 years
Osteoblastoma	• *Features* – age 10-25, dull nightly pain not relieved by NSAIDs. Vertebrate (sacrum) #1 site > femur/tibia. Mass, stiffness or limp. • *Xray* – round/ovoid osteolytic lesion (often 3-6 cm)
Osteosarcoma *#1 bony malignant tumor*	• *Features* – age 10-25, metaphysis > diaphysis, low femur/upper tibia > up femur/humerus, can cross epiphysis/joint. Mass, pain, warm. • *Xray* – large poorly marginated destructive, radiodense and lucent. "Sunburst" appearance - new bone laid down perpendicular to shaft.
	Non-Malignant (Some can become malignant)[1]
Bone cyst *Simple or Unicameral*	• *Features* – 95% involve metaphysis. Active if < 0.5 cm from physis. If > 0.5cm is latent. 50% prox humerus and 18-27% proximal femur • *Xray* - Symmetrically expansile/radiolucent with thin cortical rim. "fallen fragment" sign –fractured cortex settles to dependent cyst
Bone cyst *Aneurysmal*	• Primary neoplastic or secondary response to tumor (e.g. AVM) • *Features* – metaphysis of long bones, can be at any bone • *Xray* – eccentric location, blowout/ballooned out lesion outlined by thin subperiosteal new bone formation.
Enchondroma[1]	• *Features* – phalanx/metacarpal/tarsals > humerus/femur • *Xray* – circumscribed rarefied zone, thinning/bulging cortex, stippled
Fibrous dysplasia	• *Features* – femur, tibia, humerus (flat bones – jaw, rib, skull, not spine), ± multiple sites, endocrine (McCune-Albright syndrome) • *Xray* – elliptical central lesions mid diaphysis, sclerotic margins. If tibia involved bowing occurs (usually not with femur)
Nonossifying fibroma	• *Features* – Eccentric lesion metaphysis, may extend across large areas of long bones. Most common at distal femur, prox tibia, fibula • *Xray* – eccentric cystlike areas either uni or multiloculated. Sclerotic scalloping present along endosteal margin.
Osteo-chondroma[1]	• *Features* - Most common benign bone tumor. *Xray* – Metaphysis or diaphysis (never epiphysis) broad based or pedunculated projection. Cancellous bone & cortex blend with bone of host area.
Osteoid osteoma	• *Features* – 70-80% long bones – femur, tibia, humerus > spine > hands and feet. Age 5-20, nightly pain, relieved with NSAIDs • *Xray* –small (often < 1 cm) elliptical cortical lesions + surrounding dense sclerosis > intramedullary lesions without surrounding region.

Assessment

Disorders that Alter End Tidal CO_2 Concentrations[1]

Increasing $ETCO_2$	• *Equipment/Mechanical* – faulty exhalation valve, tourniquet release, reperfusion of an ischemic limb, transient seizure, contamination of sensor or optical bench ($\uparrow$ baseline and $ETCO_2$) • *Cardiovascular* – return of spont. circulation, $\uparrow$ cardiac output • *Pulmonary* – hypoventilation, respiratory depression, obstructive disease, rebreathing (increases baseline $ETCO_2$) • *Metabolic* – hyperthermia (including malignant), $NaHCO_3$ (onset within 1 min, lasts < 2 min.), shivering
Decreasing $ETCO_2$	• *Equipment/Mechanical* – circuit leak, partial airway obstruct, ventilator disconnection • *Cardiovascular* – cardiac arrest, shock ($\downarrow$ cardiac output), high dose epinephrine administration • *Pulmonary* – hyperventilation, bronchospasm & upper airway obstruction can $\downarrow$ steepness of respiratory upstroke – $\downarrow$ slope of waveform, mucous plugging, massive pulmonary embolism • *Metabolic* - hypothermia

[1]Assuming waveform present (if absent capnographic waveform assume dislodged ETT)

Asthma

Reference Values (PEFR[1]) for Spirometry

Age	6 years		8 years		10 years		12 years		14 years	
Sex	M[2]	F[3]	M	F	M	F	M	F	M	F
Height (in) 44	99	149	119	168	139	186	159	205	178	224
48	146	179	166	197	186	216	206	235	226	254
52	194	208	214	227	234	246	254	265	274	283
56	241	235	261	256	281	275	301	295	321	314
60	289	268	309	287	329	305	349	324	369	343
64	336	297	356	316	376	335	396	354	416	373
68	384	327	404	346	424	365	444	384	464	403
72	431	357	451	376	471	395	491	414	511	432

[1]PEFR = peak expiratory flow rate. [2]M – male, [3]F – female.

*Ann Rev Resp Dis*1983; 127: 725.

Outpatient Classification of Asthma Severity[1]

Step 1 Mild intermittent	• ≤ 5 y: symptoms ≤ 2 days/week, ≤ 2 nights/week • > 5 y: above & ≥ 80% best PEFR & < 20% variability PEFR
Step 2 Mild persistent	• ≤ 5 y: symptoms > 2X/week, but < 1X/day or > 2 nights/mo • > 5 y: above & ≥ 80% best PEFR & 20-30% variability
Step 3 Mod. persistent	• ≤ 5 y: daily symptoms, > 1 night per week • > 5 y: above & PEFR 60-80% and > 30% PEFR variability
Step 4 Severe persist	• ≤ 5 y: continual day symptoms, frequent night symptoms • > 5 y: above, PEFR 60% predicted & > 30% PEFR variability

[1]The presence of any feature is sufficient to place in higher category.

General Guidelines for Outpatient Asthma Maintenance

Step 1 Mild intermittent	• No daily medicines OR prn short acting OR oral β_2 adrenergic agonist that generally should not exceed 2 treatments/week
Step 2 Mild persistent	• Daily low dose (84-336 µg/day of beclomethasone CFC equivalent) inhaled steroids (preferred) daily OR anti-inflammatory medication (cromolyn or nedocromil) OR leukotriene antagonist (e.g. montelukast if ≥ 2 years or zafirlukast if ≥ 5 years)
Step 3 Moderate persistent	• Preferred: low to medium dose inhaled corticosteroids (< 672 µg/day of beclomethasone CFC equivalent). Alternatives include increasing inhaled steroids within medium dose range OR low to medium dose inhaled steroids with leukotriene antagonist (e.g. montelukast if ≥ 2 years or zafirlukast if ≥ 5 years) • If needed add long acting inhaled β_2-agonist or theophylline
Step 4 Severe persistent	• High dose (> 672 µg/day beclomethasone CFC equivalent) inhaled steroids AND long acting inhaled β_2-agonist (bitoterol *Tornalate*, salmeterol *Serevent*, or formeterol *Foradil* • Systemic steroids (2mg/kg/day) may be added when needed and tapered to lowest possible dose when control achieved
All Patients	• Short acting bronchodilators as needed for symptoms • ≤ 3 treatments q 20 min or a single nebulizer treated as needed • Course of systemic steroids may be needed • Use of short acting inhaled β_2-agonist on a daily basis or increasing use indicates the need to initiate or increase long term control therapy • Refer all step 4 care patients to asthma specialist. Consider referral if step 3 care required.

Theophylline has been recommended at step 3 & 4, side effects have limited its use.
Pediatr Pulmonol 2000; 29: 46. & NIH/NHLBI. Publication # 97-4051, 1997; # 02-5075, 2002

Severity of Acute Asthma Exacerbation (NIH 1997)

Feature	Mild	Moderate	Severe	Pre-Arrest
Breathless	walking	talking	at rest	
Position	can lie down	prefers sitting	sits upright	
Talking	sentences	phrases	words	
Alertness	may be agitated	usually agitated	usually agitated	drowsy/confused
Respiratory rate	Increased	Increased	rapid	
Acc. muscles	usually not	common	usually	
Wheeze	end expiratory	all expiration	insp.+expiratory	absent wheeze
Pulse	normal	elevated	elevated	bradycardia
Pulsus para.	< 10 mm Hg	10-20 mm Hg	20-40 mm Hg	may be absent
PEFR	> 80%	50-80%	< 50%	
PaO_2 room air	normal	> 60 mm Hg	< 60 mm Hg	
$PaCO_2$	< 42 mm Hg	< 42 mm Hg	$\geq$ 42 mm Hg	
O_2 sat. room air	> 95%	91-95%	< 91%	

Ann Emerg Med 1998; 31: 579.

Preschool Respiratory Assessment Measure [PRAM] ($\leq$ 6 years old)

Signs	0	1	2	3
Suprasternal retractions	Absent	-	Present	-
Scalene muscle contraction	Absent	-	Present	-
Air entry	Normal	Diminished at bases	Widespread decrease	Absent or Minimal
Wheezing	Absent	Expiratory	Inspiratory and Expiratory	Audible without stethoscope/silent chest with minimal air entry
O_2 saturation	$\geq$ 95%	92-94%	< 92%	

[1] Total score < 5 = mild airway obstruction, 5-8 = moderate airway obstruction, and $\geq$ 9 = severe airway obstruction, meaningful improvement is $\geq$ 3 change from baseline.
[2] If asymmetric findings, the most severe side is rated   *J Pediatr 2000; 137: 62.*

Criteria associated with severe disease and high likelihood of admission to hospital	• Pretreatment PEFR and FEV1 < 25% predicted • Pulsus paradoxicus > 10 mm Hg on presentation • Failure of PEFR to rise > 15% after treatment • Posttreatment PEFR and FEV1 < 60% predicted or PO_2 <60-80, PCO_2 > 40-45, pH <7.35, or SaO_2 <93%

Guidelines for ED Management of Asthma
(National Institutes of Health 1997)

History, examination, O_2 saturation, peak flow (PEFR) or FEV1

FEV1 or PEFR > 50%
- β_2 agonist by MDI or neb. X 3 1st hr
- O_2 to keep sat. $\geq$ 90 %
- Oral steroids if no immediate response

FEV1 or PEFR < 50%
- High dose β_2 agonist + anticholinergic neb q 20 min or continue X 1 hr
- O_2 to keep sat. $\geq$ 90 %
- Oral steroids

Impending arrest
- Intubation + ventilate with 100%
- β_2 agonist + anticholinergic neb.
- IV steroids

Repeat exam, PEFR, O_2 saturation as needed

Admit to ICU (see below)

Moderate exacerbation
- PEFR 50-80% of predicted best
- Moderate symptoms
- Inhaled β_2 agonists q 60 minutes
- Oral or increased inhaled steroids
- Treat 1-3 hours, if improvement

Severe exacerbation
- PEFR < 50% of predicted best
- Severe rest symptoms, high risk
- No improvement after initial treatment
- Inhaled β_2 agonists q hr or continuous + inhaled anticholinergics
- O_2 and systemic steroids

Good response
- PEFR $\geq$ 70%, sustain response 60 minutes
- Normal exam

Incomplete response
- PEFR $\geq$ 50% , < 70%
- Mild to moderate symptoms

Poor response
- PEFR < 50%
- $pCO_2 \geq$ 42 mm Hg
- Severe symptoms

OR ↓ (individualize)

Discharge home
- Continue inhaled β_2 agonists + oral steroid
- Patient education regarding medicines, review plan, follow-up

Admit to hospital
- Inhaled β_2 agonist and anticholinergic
- Oral or IV steroid
- O_2 to keep sat. $\geq$ 90 %
- Follow PEFR,HR,O_2sat

Admit to ICU
- Inhaled β_2 agonist hourly or continuous
- IV steroids
- Oxygen
- Possible intubation

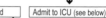

NIH Guidelines for Diagnosis/Management of Asthma *Ann Emerg Med* 1998; 31: 579.

Parenteral Agents for Treating Acute Asthma

Agent	Dose (max dose)	Frequency	Comments
epinephrine 1:1000	0.01 mg/kg SC (0.4ml)	q 20 minutes	nonselective α, β agonist
Sus-Phrine 1:200	0.005 ml/kg SC (0.2ml)	single dose	long acting epinephrine
ketamine	1-2 mg/kg IV	-	for intubated patients
magnesium sulfate	25-50 mg/kg IV (2 g)	-	administer over 15 min
methylprednisolone	1-2 mg/kg IV	q 6 hours	-
terbutaline (1mg/ml)	0.01 mg/kg SC	q 20 minutes	more β selective than epi
terbutaline	2 µg/kg IV over 5min then 4.5 µg /kg/h	load over 5 min 4.5 µg/kg/hour	monitor in ICU , reduce dose 50% if theophylline

Inhaled Asthma Medications

Agent	Dose/Frequency[1]	Comments
albuterol 0.05% (Ventolin)	Neb: 0.5-1ml q30min or continuous, then 2 puffs q 4h (MDI)	β agonist (more selective β_2 than isoetharine, and metaproterenol)
atropine (1mg/ml)	0.03-0.05 ml/kg q30 minX2	more tachycardia than β agonists
beclomethasone (Vanceril)	1-2 puffs tid-qid	not approved < 6 yr
cromolyn (Intal)	Neb: 20 mg tid-qid or 2 puffs tid-qid (MDI)	maintenance only, ± not useful acutely
flunisolide(Aerobid)	2 puffs bid (MDI)	not approved < 6 y
ipratropium (Atrovent)	Neb: 250 µg q 6-8h 1-2 puffs qid (MDI)	anticholinergic with longer onset of action than most β agonists
isoetharine 1% (Bronkosol)	Neb: 0.25-0.5 ml q 20 min, then q 4-6 h	poor β_2 selectivity
metaproterenol (Alupent)	0.25-.5 mg/kg/dose q4-6 h	less β_2 selective, max dose 15 mg
salmeterol (Serevent)	1-2 puffs qid (MDI)	long acting β maintenance, >11 y

[1]Nebulizer (mixed with 2.5 ml NS) unless otherwise stated, MDI - metered dose inhaler.

Oral Asthma Medications

Agent	Preparation	Dose	Comment
albuterol (Ventolin)	2 mg/5ml Tabs: 2,4 mg	0.10-0.15 mg/kg per dose (tid-qid)	β agonist
metaproterenol (Alupent)	10 mg/5ml Tabs: 10, 20 mg	2 mg/kg/day (qid)	β agonist
montelukast (Singulair) [leukotriene inhibitor]	Tabs: 4, 5, 10 mg	4 mg qhs 2-5 y 5 mg qhs 6-14 y 10 mg qhs > 14 y	prophylactic, not for acute treatment
prednisolone-Pediapred 5/5 Prelone & Orapred 15/5	15 mg/5ml; 5 mg/5ml Tabs: 5 mg	1-2 mg/kg/day	steroid, if treat 5-7 d no taper needed
prednisone (LiquidPred)	5 mg/5ml; Tabs: 1, 2.5, 5, 10, 20, 50	1-2 mg/kg/day	" "
zafirlukast (Accolate) [leukotriene antagonist]	Tabs: 10, 20 mg	10 mg bid 5-11 y 20 mg bid > 11 y	prophylactic, not for acute treatment

Bronchiolitis

Bronchiolitis is a lung infection that commonly occurs in infants ≤ 8 months old with most cases occurring during the winter. Respiratory syncytial virus (RSV) causes 60-90% of cases followed by other viruses, Mycoplasma & Chlamydia. The median duration of symptoms is 12 days with 18% ill at 21 and 9% still ill at 28 days.

Risk Factors for Severe Disease/Respiratory Failure in < 1 Year Old[1]

• Ill or toxic appearance	• Gestational age < 34 weeks
• Oxygen saturation < 95%	• Atelectasis on CXR
• Respiratory rate ≥ 70 breaths/min	• Age < 3 months

Single best predictor of severe disease may be ↓ oxygen saturation (esp. with feeding)
Am J Dis Child 1991; 145: 151.

Evidence Based Hospital Management Guidelines for Bronchiolitis
Excluding children > 1 year or with prior wheezing episode

Overview	• Keep patient well hydrated and oxygenated
Monitoring	• Cardiac and pulse oximetry – discontinue electric monitoring in timely manner to help transition to home
Labs/Xrays	• Routine NP swab for RSV not indicated - may be used for isolation of select patients and for identification of patients at high risk for resp. failure (e.g. congenital heart disease [CHD], pulm HTN, bronchopulmonary dysplasia [BPD]) • CXR not recommended as routine
Respiratory care	• **Not recommended** – chest physiotherapy, cool mist, saline aerosol, inhaled steroids, routine bronchodilators • **Recommended** – epinephrine inhalation, 0.5 mg of 0.1% solution (0.5 ml in 3.5 ml of NS) in select patients. If not better within 60 min., do not repeat. If better may repeat. • *Oxygen if < 93% saturation or respiratory distress* • *Although their use is controversial, a meta-analysis showed that steroids (prednisone/prednisolone 1 mg/kg/d) may lead to improved symptoms, ↓ length of hospitalization & symptom. Pediatrics 2000; 105: 106*
Isolation	• Respiratory/contact isolation
Discharge criteria	• Resp rate < 80 (*preferably lower*) - room air or < 0.5 L/min • O₂ saturation > 93% on room air. • Patient is taking oral feedings without difficulty • Patient on oral or regularly administered agents • Adequate home support, Dr. notified/follow up.

Palivizumab (*Synagis*) 15 mg/kg IM q month of RSV season or RSV Immune globulin are used prophylactically if premature (< 32 weeks gestation X 6 mo; < 28 weeks X 12 mo) or with BPD until 2 years old. Ribavirin use is controversial ± if severe disease, cystic fibrosis, CHD, premie, BPD. *Pediatrics*1999;104:1334;& 1998;102:1211;& 2000;105:e44.

Cystic Fibrosis

Inherited defect exocrine gland secretion (1) chronic pulmonary disease, (2) malabsorption due to pancreatic insufficiency & (3)↑ sweat electrolytes with variable expression & severity of disease manifestations. Suspect based on symptoms and confirm via sweat test, ± newborn immunoreactive trypsinogen, DNA sampling.

Organ	Manifestation & Management
GI	• <u>Cholelithiasis</u> – up to 5% have stones, 5% have cholestasis, biliary cirrhosis rare. Ursodeoxycholate slows progression of liver lesions.
	• <u>DIOS – distal intestinal obstruction syndrome</u> – later in childhood, distal small bowel obstruction, pain, ↓ stooling, ± diet/med non-compliance. If incomplete, ± *Miralax*, *GoLYTELY*, lactulose.
	• <u>Meconium ileus</u> - 15% (obstruct distal small bowel with meconium) in 1st 48 h life. Hyperosmolar enemas 50% relief, others need surgery.
	• <u>Meconium plug syndrome</u> – a more benign blockage of colon.
	• <u>Rectal prolapse</u> - may be presenting symptom (esp. < 3 years)
	• <u>Pancreatic insufficiency</u> - leading to malabsorption occurs in 90% by age 1. Leads to failure to thrive and later diabetes. Enzyme replacement → adequate fat absorption in up to 80%.
Lung	• <u>Airway obstruction</u> – inhaled DNase (*Pulmozyme*) & intermittent inhaled tobramycin will↓ viscosity sputum, ↑ lung function. Bronchodilators and oral/inhaled steroids may be useful.
	• <u>Hemoptysis</u> – see management below (admit if > 30-60 ml)
	• <u>Infection</u> – Use prior cultures to guide antibiotics, obtain new cultures. S. aureus & Pseudomonas are common (may require fluoroquinolones). Antibiotics until baseline symptom status (usually ≥ 14 d). Low admit threshold – pO_2 < 60, infiltrate, atelectasis, distress
	• <u>Pneumothorax</u> develops in 5-8%, chest tube for all > 10% in size
Metabolic	• Low K, Na, Cl with alkalosis due to respiratory/sweat loss

J Pediatr 2002; 140: 156.

Grunting

Most Common Etiology of Grunting in Children Presenting to a Pediatric ED	**Cardiorespiratory**	**57%**
	Upper or lower respiratory tract infection	28%
	Reactive airway disease	20%
	Aspiration foreign body/liquid	4%
	Myocarditis, CHF, congenital heart	4%
	Sickle cell – acute chest syndrome	2%
	Nonrespiratory Infection	**25%**
	Bacteremia/sepsis	12%
	Fever, viral infection	6%
	Meningitis/pyelonephritis (4% each)	4%
Pediatr Emerg Care 1995; 11: 158.	**Surgical** abd (intussus, obstruct) or ileus	**8%**
	Sickle crisis, VP shunt malfunction, Corneal abrasion, skull fx, hemolytic anemia	2% each

Hemoptysis

Mild - < 150 ml/d; large 150-400 ml/d; massive - > 400 ml/day (variable definitions)

Etiology of Hemoptysis for Children Admitted to Hospital

Cystic fibrosis	65%	Neoplasm	3%	Nasopharyngeal	1%
Congenital heart		Pulm HTN, bleed,		Sepsis	1%
disease	15%	embolism	2%	Vasculitides	1%
Pneumonia	6%	Tuberculosis	1%	Other	5%

Overall 13% died, esp. older, ↑amount, fever, transfusion.   *Pediatrics* 1997; 100: 37.
Management - Intubate if airway compromise, type and cross blood, Administer NS, blood as needed for massive bleeding. Reverse bleeding disorder (platelets, FFP). Bronchoscopy may be required as well as bronchial artery embolization (pulmonologist and thoracic surgery/interventional radiologist consult).

Pneumonia

Bordetella pertussis mimics chlamydial pneumonitis, but has a paroxysmal, inspiratory 'whoop' (may be absent < 6 months). Prolonged coughing attacks may lead to cyanosis, emesis, anoxia. *Chlamydia* 3-16 weeks. 1st rhinorrhea, then staccato cough, ↑RR, rales or wheeze. 95% afebrile, 50% have concurrent/prior conjunctivitis. *Mycoplasma* - low-grade fever, malaise, headache, nonproductive cough lasting weeks. It is responsible for 9-21% of school-aged pneumonia, may occur in epidemics with little seasonal variation. *Pneumococcus and H flu* are typically associated with abrupt onset of high fever and dyspnea, and may be preceded by a viral URI. *Tuberculosis* subacute cough, night sweats, ↓ weight.

Age	Etiology
newborn	Causes - Group B streptococcus, E coli, Listeria, and herpes virus
1-4 months	*Febrile:* pneumococcus, H flu (rare). *Afebrile:* chlamydia, ureaplasma, mycoplasma, pneumocystis, and cytomegalovirus
5 months - 5 years	Viruses (especially RSV) are most common, followed by pneumococcus, Mycoplasma. H flu is now rare. Ratio of viral to bacterial etiology > 5:2.
>5 years	Mycoplasma followed by pneumococcus

Predictive Value of Respiratory Rate In Pneumonia	Age	Respiratory rate[1,3]	Sensitivity	NPV[2]
	0-5 months	≥ 59	83%	99%
	6-11 months	≥ 52	67%	98%
	1-2 years	≥ 42	71%	96%

[1]Breaths/min. [2]NPV – negative predictive value. [3] One study found a ↑RR in only 10% with pneumonia. Only 45% had resp. distress, rales, ↑RR or ↓breath sounds ≤ age 5.
          Arch Pediatr Adolesc Med 1995;149:283.; *Pediatr Emerg Care* 2001;17:240.

Indications for Hospital Admission

• Age < 2-3 months	• Toxic appearance
• Lobar infiltrate and < 12 months	• Immunocompromised
• Multilobar, effusion, pneumatocoele	• Unresponsive to oral medications
• Respiratory distress or hypoxia	• Unable to keep down liquids or meds

Antibiotic therapy for pneumonia is detailed on page 81.

Stridorous Upper Airway Diseases in Children

Feature	Croup	Bacterial Tracheitis	Epiglottitis	Retropharyngeal Abscess
Age (y)	0.3-3.0	5-10	2-8	Median 3.5
Prodrome	days	hours -days	Min-hours	days (prior URI)
Fever	low grade	usual	usual	usual
Xray[1]	steeple sign[1]	exudate	Ratios[2]	soft tissue swelling[3]
Etiology	viral	*S. aureus*	*H. influenzae*	Strep/Staph/anaerobe
Cough	yes	yes	no	uncommon
Drool	no	no	yes	yes
Toxic	no	yes	yes	yes
Antibiotics	no	yes	yes	yes

[1] Do not rely on soft tissue lateral neck Xrays exclusively to diagnose or exclude most disorders. In epiglottitis, films are read as normal up to 60%. In croup, films are read as normal in 50%, epiglottitis in 20% and croup in only 30%. *Laryngoscope* 1985; 95:1159.
[2] 3 calculations reported as 100% sensitive/highly specific for epiglottitis: AEW/C3W>.35, EW/C3W>0.50, & EW/C3W>0.6: *EW=epiglottic width, EH=epiglottic height, C3W= C3 vertebral width, and AEW=aryepiglottic fold width.* *Ann Emerg Med* 1990; 19: 978
[3] Retropharynx soft tissue > 7 mm ant. to C2, > 14 mm ant. to C5/6. (CT is more accurate)

Croup Score (add the 5 elements together)[1]

Feature	0	1	2	3
Color	normal	dusky	cyanotic	cyanotic on O_2
Air movement	normal	mild↓	moderate↓	marked↓
Retractions	none	mild	moderate	severe
Mentation	normal	restless	lethargic	obtunded
Stridor	none	mild	moderate	severe/obstructed

Total score	Severity	Treatment
0-4	mild	cool mist, home care
5-6	mild/moderate	cool mist, admit if <6 months or unreliable family
7-8	moderate	racemic epinephrine, consider steroids, admit most
9-14	severe	racemic epinephrine, steroids, ICU admission
15	terminal	racemic epinephrine, steroids, intubation

[1] Any category with score of 3, classify as severe. *Taussig: Am J Dis Child* 1975; 129: 790.

Croup Management

- **Humidified** O_2 (recent study found mist to be ineffective in moderate croup.)[1]
- **Dexamethasone** 0.6 mg/kg IM or 0.15-0.6 mg/kg PO, or oral prednisolone (1-2 mg/kg/d X 1-3 days)
- **Aerosolized racemic epinephrine** (RE) 0.25-0.50 ml of 2.25% solution diluted 1:8 or standard epinephrine 1 ml of 1:1,000 (cheaper + similar side effects). Improved children treated with RE with no worsening in 3h may be discharged.
- **Aerosolized budesonide** – 2 mg (4 ml) via nebulizer
- **Heliox** – when inhaled may be useful at decreasing airway resistance.
[1] *Acad Emerg Med* 2002; 9: 488.

Reye's Syndrome

Overview: 70% with Reye's syndrome have had recent URI (e.g., influenza A or B), 15-30% recent varicella, and 2-15% recent diarrhea. Most cases occur during peak influenza period of January to March. 0.05% patients with influenza B + 0.003% with influenza A develop Reye's. Reye's is associated with isopropyl alcohol, lead, methyl bromide, insecticides, insect repellent, aflatoxin, phenothiazines, and aspirin use. Patients develop inflammation & edema of liver & brain.

Clinical Features
- Vomiting 1 week after prodromal illness
- Headache, lethargy, seizures (30%)
- Absent meningeal signs
- Younger children (less vomiting, less prodrome)
- Hepatomegaly (within 24-48 hours of diagnosis)

Clinical Stage	Signs and Symptoms
0	alert, vomiting, liver dysfunction
I	lethargic, vomiting, liver dysfunction
II	delirious, combative
III	obtunded, decorticate, reactive pupils, possible seizures
IV	obtunded, decerebrate, unreactive pupils
V	flaccid, areflexic, apneic, liver function often normalized

Labs in Reye's Syndrome	Treatment of Reye's Syndrome

• ↑ AST/ALT (≥ 2X normal) - most sensitive screening test
• ↑ ammonia (≥ 1.5 normal) - rises early and normalizes quickly
• → bilirubin (< 3 mg/dl)
• ↓ glucose (70-80% of infants)
• ↓pCO₂, ↓CO₂
• ↑creatinine and↑BUN in 30-40%
• ↑amylase (pancreatitis in 9%)
	• D₁₀.9NS keep glucose150-200 mg/dl
	• Keep fluids at 2/3 maintenance rate
	• If ≥ Stage II consider:
	  - intubation, elevate head of bed (all III, and II if ammonia > 300)
	  - deep sedation
	  - cerebral pressure monitoring
	  - mannitol 0.5-1 g/kg IV q 6 h
	  - lactulose 0.3g/kg PO/NG q 6 h

Prognosis: Risk of progression from stage I to coma is high with ↑ transaminases, PT (>3 seconds above normal), or ammonia (>100 µg/dl). Poor prognosis at stage II-IV level is indicated by age < 1 year, ammonia 6 X normal, CK 10 X normal, rapid progression, or seizures in stage III. Most recover without sequelae. 10% develop chronic neurologic problems (e.g., seizure disorder, encephalopathy).

Uniform Reporting & Outcomes for Submersion Injury

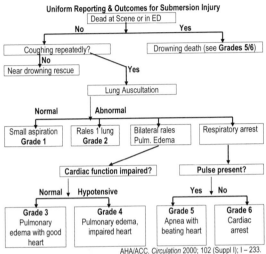

AHA/ACC. *Circulation* 2000; 102 (Suppl I); I – 233.

Clinical Grade and Submersion Mortality

Grade	Definition	Mortality
1	Normal auscultation with coughing	0%
2	Abnormal lung exam with rales in some fields	0.6%
3	Acute pulmonary edema, no arterial hypotension	5.2%
4	Acute pulmonary edema, with arterial hypotension	19.4%
5	Isolated respiratory arrest	44%
6	Cardiopulmonary arrest	93%

AHA/ACC. *Circulation* 2000; 102 (Suppl I); I – 233.

Factors Associated with High Mortality Following Submersion

Factor	Mortality	Factor	Mortality
• Submersion > 25 min	100%	• Fixed pupils in ED	89%
• CPR > 25 min	100%	• Severe acidosis in ED	89%
• Pulseless on ED arrival	100%	• Respiratory arrest on	
• VF/VT on 1st monitor	93%	ED arrival	87%

AHA/ACC. *Circulation* 2000; 102 (Suppl I); I – 233.

Surgical Abdominal Disorders

Most Common Etiologies of Abdominal Pain in Children Presenting to a Pediatric ED *Pediatr Emerg Care 1992;8:126*	Nonspecific pain	36%	Pharyngitis	6%
	Gastroenteritis	16%	Viral illness	3%
	Appendicitis	8%	Pneumonia	2%
	Constipation	7%	Otitis Media	2%
	Urinary infection	6%	Other disease	14%

High Yield Criteria for Ordering Plain Abd. Xrays in Children	The presence any criteria is 93-100% sensitive in detecting plain Xrays that are
• prior abdominal surgery, • peritoneal signs, • foreign body ingestion, • abdominal distention, or • abnormal bowel sounds	diagnostic or suggestive of major surgical disease. If no criteria are present, plain films have < 1% probability of revealing a surgical disorder. Plain films are normal in 50% and misleading in 2% with surgical disease.

Ann Emerg Med 1992; 21:1423.

Radiologic Studies in Surgical Abdominal Disorders

Disorder	Radiologic adjunct	Key features
Appendicitis	Ultrasound	Multiple pediatric studies with sensitivity of 80-90%. Less accurate if perforated/gangrenous
	Computerized tomography	90% sensitive without contrast, up to 98-100% sensitive with rectal contrast. May be less useful in younger patients with less fat.
Hirschprung's	Barium enema	Shows normal rectum, dilated proximal colon
Intussusception	Ultrasound	98% sensitive in limited studies
	Barium or air contrast enema	Air contrast enema is standard for diagnosis with 60-90% successful reduction rate
Meckel's	Technetium scan	95% sensitive (esp. if given with cimetidine) False negatives occur if little gastric mucosa
Malrotation	Ultrasonography	May show bowel wall edema, intraluminal fluid
	UGI series	Shows obstruction at 3rd portion duodenum
Pyloric stenosis	Ultrasound	89-95% sensitive
	UGI series	95% sensitive, risks aspiration, delays surgery

Pediatr Emerg Med Reports 1997; 2: 111.

Appendicitis

Frequency of Historical Features at Different Ages

0-2 years (rare)		2-5 years (< 5% all cases)		6-12 years	
Vomiting	85-90%	Abdominal Pain	89-100%	Pain	98%
Pain	35-77%	Vomiting (*unlike*	66-100%	↑ with move	41-75%
Fever	40-60%	*older children*		Vomiting	68-95%
Diarrhea	18-46%	*& adults,*		*before pain*	≤ 18%
Irritability	35-40%	*vomiting may*		Anorexia	47-75%
Cough/rhinitis	40%	*precede pain)*		Diarrhea	9-16%
Grunting	8-23%	Fever	80-87%	Constipation	5-28%
Hip pain/stiff	3-23%	Anorexia	53-60%	Dysuria	4-20%

Frequency of Physical Exam Features at Different Ages

Temp > 100 F	87-100%	Temp > 100 F	82%	Temp > 100.4F	
Diffuse tender	55-92%	RLQ tender	58-85%	< 24 hours	4%
RLQ tender	< 50%	Diffuse tender	19-28%	> 24 hours	64%
Distention	30-52%	Invol. Guarding	85%	RLQ tender	>80-95%
Lethargy	40%	Rebound tender	50%	Diffuse tender	15%
Mass	30%			Rebound	~ 50%

Risk of Appendicitis
MANTRELS scoring system[1]

Total	Action
≥ 7	Candidates for surgery
4-6	Serial exams or further testing (CT or US)
< 4	Extremely low probability of appendicitis

Item	Score
Migration of pain to RLQ	1
Anorexia or acetone in urine	1
Nausea with vomiting	1
Tenderness in right low quadrant	2
Rebound tenderness	1
Elevated temperature > 100.4 F	1
Leukocytosis; WBC > 10,500	2
Shift of WBC's; >75% neutrophils	1

[1] This score is underlined in younger children & infants.

- WBC count (↑ in as few as 18% < 24hours & up to 90% ≥ 48 hour of symptoms)
- UA – 7-24% have > 5 WBC or RBCs/HPF
- Ultrasound – 80-90% sensitive (diameter > 6 mm, target sign, wall > 2 mm)
- CT - > 95% sensitive (esp. if 5 mm cuts, using colonic contrast) – Fat streaking, > 6 mm appendix, focal cecal apical thickening are most common CT findings. (in very young, smaller appendix, less fat amount/streaking may ↓ CT accuracy)

Ann Emerg Med 2000; 36: 39.

Annular pancreas is associated with malrotation and Downs syndrome. Bilious vomiting is the hallmark, as the obstruction is distal to the Ampulla of Vater.

Gastric volvulus A torsion ≤ 180 degrees produces a partial obstruction with or without vomiting which may not lead to vascular compromise. Torsion > 180 degrees causes Borchardt's triad: (1) retching, (2) acute epigastric pain, (3) distention with inability to pass a NG. Respiratory distress or GI bleeding occur.

Hirschsprung's Disease (congenital megacolon): Congenital absence of parasympathetic ganglion cells in Auerbach's plexus (myenteric) and Meissner's (submucosal) plexus in the intestine, causing un-coordinated intestinal motility. In 80-90%, involvement is limited to rectum and rectosigmoid colon including the internal anal sphincter. Hirschsprung's is noted in 1/5,000 births and is more common in males and Down's syndrome. In newborns, it may present as complete obstruction or delayed passage of meconium with mild constipation. Most affected infants are full term. If left untreated, failure to thrive will be noted, with ill appearance, malnourishment, or chronic constipation. The most serious complication is the development of ulcerative enterocolitis, which may be lethal. In this complication, elevated luminal pressures in the proximal normal colon inhibit total colonic blood flow and shunt blood away from the mucosa. Bowel wall edema, mucosal necrosis and sepsis occur. Diagnosis is made by barium enema (BE). If BE is nondiagnostic, consider rectal biopsy with acetylcholinesterase histochemistry on mucosa and submucosal biopsy specimens. Children with functional constipation are generally healthy appearing with bowel troubles beginning around age 2 years or the time of toilet training, have stool in rectal vault, & fecal soiling. Hirschsprung's patients are generally younger, have empty rectal vault, and no fecal soiling.

Incarcerated hernias Manual reduction may be useful regardless of time and may still work if obstruction is present. Avoid manual reduction if peritonitis, unstable vitals, significant erythema or other sign of strangulation. Bimanual abdominal/rectal exam may identify mass between fingers, a finding absent in spermatic cord hydrocele. Palpation of the inguinal region may reveal a dilated external ring or a silk glove sign (smoothness felt as if 2 pieces of silk are being rubbed together when rolling the spermatic cord in a direction perpendicular to the inguinal canal).

Intussusception Telescoping of 1 intestinal segment into another, the #1 cause of obstruction from 3 mo to 6 y. Mean age is 8 mo, with 80% < 2 y. Origin unknown in 90% unless < 1 mo or > 3 y where lead point (e.g., tumor) may be found.

Predisposing Conditions
• Henoch Schonlein Purpura (HSP) is noted in 3% of cases. None are reducible.
• Cystic fibrosis - Barium enema reduction is unlikely in cystic fibrosis.
• Peutz Jehgers syndrome is a rare cause of intussusception in older children.
• Intestinal lymphosarcoma can cause chronic non-strangulating intussusception and should be suspected in all cases of intussusception older than 6 years.
• Post-operative - after retroperitoneal dissection (e.g., Wilm's tumor).

Clinical features: A previously well infant who paroxysmally cries out, draws up legs & vomits. Passage of a formed/liquid stool provides relief with recurrence in 20-60 min. Child may be lethargic. Exam may reveal distention and/or a sausage shaped mass, in RUQ. Independent predictors include highly suggestive Xray (mass, visible intussusceptum, obstruction; (Odds Ratio [OR] – 18), rectal bleed (OR – 17), vomit (OR – 13), & male (OR – 6). It is estimated that 84-100% have at least one of these features. *Arch Pediatr Adoles Med* 2000; 154: 252.

Diagnosis/Treatment: Plain X-rays are definitive in as few as 21% of cases with 53% read as equivocal and 26% as normal with radiologists agreeing on Xray diagnosis in as few as 10-15%.

Plain Abdominal X-ray findings[1]			
	Sparse large bowel gas	63%	Target sign[2]	63%
	Sparse cecal feces	70%	Crescent sign[3]	30%
	Small bowel obstruction	42%	Cecal gas visible	10%
	Soft tissue mass	42%	Cecal feces visible	3%

[1] Soft tissue mass & sparse large bowel gas are best predictors of intussusception (likelihood ratios [LR] of 3.9 & 2.5), while visible cecal gas [LR - 0.25], and visible cecal feces [LR – 0.11] are the best predictors of not having intussusception. Importantly - all of listed Xray findings were found in those with and without intussusception.
[2] *Target sign* - outer ring of fat density, & concentric inner fat density ring to right of spine
[3] *Crescent sign* - soft tissue mass of intussusceptum projecting into transverse colon
Pediatr Radiol 1992; 22: 110. & 1994; 24: 17.

US may be diagnostic with classic "bulls eye" appearance in > 95%. BE or air-contrast enema reduces 60-90%. An enema is often therapeutic but should be avoided if shock, peritoneal signs, perforation, or high grade obstruction.

Protocol for Air or Contrast Reduction of Intussusception
• Consult surgeon, place NG, fluid resuscitation, prepare OR.
• Insert non-lubricated 20-24F Foley into rectum, inflate balloon 5-10 ml and pull down against levators. Compress buttocks and tape together, wrap legs.
• Allow contrast agent to flow by gravity into colon from height of <1 meter.
• Stop attempt if contrast column is stationary and outline unchanged for 10 min.
• DO NOT palpate abdomen during procedure and use fluoroscope intermittently.
• Reduction is complete when there is (1) free flow of barium or air into small bowel, (2) expulsion of feces and flatus with contrast, (3) disappearance of mass, or (4) improvement in the child's condition.

Malrotation and Midgut Volvulus. Malrotation includes a wide spectrum of congenital anomalies of incomplete rotation of the intestine during fetal development. Symptoms occur due to volvulus, duodenal compression by Ladd bands or other adhesive bands affecting the small and large intestine. 25-50% of adolescents are asymptomatic. Volvulus (one emergency complication occurring in 30% with malrotation) characterized by sudden vomiting which may be bilious bloody or coffee ground. Stool often contains blood. *J Pediatr Surg* 2000; 35: 756.

Presenting Features of Midgut Volvulus			
At diagnosis, age < 1 week	24%	Plain radiographs	
age < 3-4 weeks	64-75%	gastric/duodenal distention	
age < 6 months	86%	*(double bubble sign – also*	
Vomiting (bilious in 77%)	100%	*found in duodenal atresia)*	
Diarrhea	23%	gas paucity after duodenum	
Bloody stool	17%	UGI series diagnostic	94-100%
Abdominal distention	43%	(86% specific)	
Normal abdominal exam	36%	Barium enema diagnostic	81%
Features in infants above 2 months old with malrotation included bilious vomiting in 49%, nonbilious vomiting in 49%, pain in 31%, failure to thrive in 23%, and fever 23%			
Management			

- Fluid resuscitation (NS 20 ml/kg IV, repeat as needed), NG tube to suction
- Broad spectrum antibiotics (esp. perforation) – see page 77, 81.
- Surgical consultation
- UGI series if stable (if perforation or obstruction, may need immediate surgery)

*ClinPerinatology*1996;23:353; *WorldJSurg*1993;17:326; *JPediatrSurg*1989;24:777.

Meckel's diverticulum arises from failure of omphalomesenteric duct to close. It is found in 2% of the population within 2 feet (100 cm) of the ileocecal valve. Most individuals remain asymptomatic, with complications developing at some point in 23-40%. Complications usually occur prior to 10-30 years of age. Obstruction is most common presentation if intussusception is also present. Bleeding can be the major manifestation, especially in children < 2 years old. Meckel's account for 50% of lower GI bleeding in this age range. Bleeding is usually painless and sudden. Inflammation (e.g. diverticulitis) may present like appendicitis in 20%, and is most common around age 8 years. Up to 50% perforate before surgery. Diagnosis of Meckel's is made with a Technetium (Tc99 or "Meckel's") scan, which has a sensitivity of 75-100% and a specificity of 80%. A higher incidence of true positives occur if cimetidine is given 24h prior to the scan, if the clinical condition permits this delay. By blocking histamine, cimetidine prevents secretion and increases concentration of Tc from gastric mucosa. BE is only diagnostic in 4-20% of cases.

Necrotizing enterocolitis primarily in premature infants and is occasionally diagnosed later. Mean age is 6-7 d, rare cases > 100 d. 55% < 1.5 kg at birth.

Modified Bell Staging Criteria for NEC			
Stage/Classification	Systemic signs	Bowel signs	Xray signs
IA suspected NEC	Temp. unstable, apnea, ↓ HR	↑ pregavage residual, distend, vomit, heme +	Normal or dilation or ileus
IB suspected NEC	See above	Rectal bleeding	See above
IIA proven NEC (mildly ill)	See above	IB + absent bowel sounds, ± tender	Ileus, pneumatosis intestinalis
IIB proven NEC (moderately ill)	Above, + mild met. acidosis, ↓ platelets	Above ± abdomen cellulitis, RLQ mass	Above portal gas, ± ascites
IIIA advanced NEC (critical/no perf.)	IIB plus ↓ BP, ↓ HR, apnea, DIC, ↓WBC	Above + peritonitis, tender, distention	Above + definite ascites
IIIB advanced NEC (critical/perforation)	See IIIA	See IIIA	IIB + pneumoperitoneum

Strictures develop in 11-36% of NEC cases, and may result in or bowel obstruction. *Treatment* – (1) place NG, and administer IV fluids, ± albumin 1 g/kg q 6-8 h. TPN often needed. (2) IV ampicillin & gentamicin, + vancomycin if *S. epidermidis* is prominent in NICU or + cultures, & clindamycin or *Flagyl* if perforation. See pg 77,81 for dose, (3) blood to keep Hct 35-40%, (4) ventilator, (5) inotropes (6) Xrays q 6-8 hours to R/O perf. (7) surgery indications: pneumoperitoneum, intestinal gangrene ± clinical deteriorate, portal vein gas, abd. wall cellulitis, fixed mass.

Pyloric Stenosis (PS) in 1/3,000 infants, males > females. PS is rare in premature and more common in 1st born males, ↑ maternal age. 21% have urinary tract anomalies. Symptoms begin at 2-3 weeks, PS can be seen up to 5 mo.

Clinical features: Non-bilious vomit during/after feeding, projectile vomiting over ensuing week. Patients are hungry with poor weight gain. *Physical Examination:* Abdomen - peristaltic waves or a palpable "olive" in 33-53% (# from prospective studies, lower than classically taught). Hypochloremic metabolic alkalosis.

Diagnosis/Management: Algorithm places infants into high/low risk categories.

Volumetric Method for Imaging Nonbilious Vomiting in Infancy	
Step 1	• Fluid resuscitation as needed, measure/correct electrolyte problems
Step 2	• NPO status 3-4 hours pre-assessment
Step 3	• Place #8 feeding tube measure volume of stomach contents
≥ 5 ml aspirate	• 91% sensitive for pyloric stenosis, at this point consult surgery • if surgeon palpates olive, surgery may be indicated without imaging • If no olive palpated, perform US, • If + US perform surgery, If US negative, perform UGI series • If + UGI series, perform surgery, if negative treat medically
< 5 ml aspirate	• Only 12% probability of pyloric stenosis, perform UGI series • If positive, surgery, if negative treat medically

Pediatrics 1999; 103: 1198., *Pediatr Radiol* 1997; 27: 175-177.

Ultrasonography (≥ 4 mm pyloric muscle thickness or ≥ 14 mm length) and UGI series are > 90-95% sensitive for diagnosing pyloric stenosis.

Identification of Abused Drug Based on Street Name

Street name	Drug[1]	Street name	Drug[1]	Street name	Drug[1]
1 & 1	T + tri, T + Rit, Rit + V,	Jamestown	Jimsonweed	Shrooms	Psilocybe
		Jet	Ketamine	Silent partnr	Heroin
Acid	LSD	John Hinckly	PCP	Sinsemilla	Marijuana
Angel dust	LSD	Joy stick	MJ + PCP	Smack	Heroin
Apples	MJ	Juice	PCP	Snow-candy	Cocaine
Bam	H + Preludin	Junk	Heroin	Snort/nuff	Cocaine
Bazooka	Cocaine	Ketamine		Special LA	Ketamine
Bazooka paste	MJ+procaine	green/purpl	LSD	Speckld bird	Lookalike A
Bennies	A	Lady	Cocaine	Speed	A or M
Black beauty	CaffeinePPA	Loads	Cod + glu	Speedball	H + C
Black Molly	lookalike A	Love (ly)	PCP	Stardust	Cocaine
Blue Angels	A	Loveboat	MJ + PCP	Stuff	Heroin
Boat	PCP	Mauve	Ketamine	Super grass	PCP
Breakin'	Heroin	Maze	Fentanyl	SuperC or K	Ketamine
Brick	MJ	Mex. Maid	Heroin	Syrup&bean	Cod + V
Butt Naked	PCP	Mcky Mouse	LSD	T's & Blues	T + tri
Chiva	HMB	Monster	M	T's & Purple	T/tri/Narcan
Christmas trees	Depressant or stimulant	Mr. Natural	LSD	Tar	Opium
		Mud	H/molasses	Thriller	Heroin
Clickers	MJ + PCP	NASA	Heroin	Tic & Tac	PCP
Coast	Ritalin IV	Newboy	Heroin	Toot	Cocaine
Coke (Cola)	Cocaine	Nose candy	Cocaine	Tootsie roll	HMB
Crack	Rock C	Packs	Cod + glu	Tolley	Toluene
Crank	A, H, or M	Pasta	Cocaine	Unicorn	LSD
Crystal	M	Perks	Percdan/cet	USDA	Heroin
Disco hits	PCP	Peruvnwhite	Cocaine	Vitamin C	Cocaine
Dishrag	Heroin	Persia white	Fentanyl	WACs	MJ/blackflag roach killer
Dollies	Methadone	Pink & Grey	Darvon		
Dust (ed)	PCP	Pinkhearts	Lookalike A	Wack	PCP
Eve	Ecstasy	President	Heroin	Watergate	Heroin
4 & doors	Cod + glu	Purple	Ketamine	West Coast	Rit IV
Footballs	A	Risking high	Heroin	Whippet	Nitrousoxide
Girl	Cocaine	Robin's egg	Lookalike A	White(dust)	Cocaine
Green	Ketamine	Rock	A or M	White, China	Fentanyl
Happy dust	Cocaine	Roofies	Flunitrazepm	Window	
Happy sticks	MJ + PCP	Scat/Skag	Heroin	pane	LSD
Hawaiian wood rose	PCP	Shermans/ Sherms	PCP + MJ or formaldhyd	Wizard	LSD
				Yo Yo	Yohimbine

[1] A (Amphetamines), C (Cocaine), Cod (codeine), glu (glutethemide), H (Heroin), Heroin – Mexican Brown (HMB), Marijuana (MJ), M (Methamphetamines), Rit (Ritalin), T (Talwin), tri (tripelennamine), V (Valium).

Toxins that Affect Vitals Signs and Physical Examination

Hypotension			Hypertension
ACE inhibitors	Antidepressants	Nitroprusside	Amphetamines
α & β antagonists	Disulfuram	Opioids	Anticholinergics
Anticholinergics	Ethanol, methanol	Organophosphate	Cocaine, Lead
Arsenic (acutely)	Iron, isopropanol	Phenothiazines	MAO inhibitors
Ca^{+2} channel block	Mercury, GHB	Sedatives	Phencyclidine
Clonidine, cyanide	Nitrates	Theophylline	Sympathomimetics

Tachycardia		Bradycardia
Amphetamines	Ethylene glycol, iron	Antidysrhythmics
Anticholinergics	Organophosphates	α agonists, β antagonists
Arsenic (acutely)	Sympathomimetics	Ca^{+2} channel blockers
Antidepressants	PCP, Phenothiazines	Digitalis, opioids, GHB
Digitalis, disulfuram	Theophylline	Organophosphates

Tachypnea		Bradypnea	
Ethylene glycol	Salicylates	Barbiturates	Isopropanol
Methanol	Sympathomimetics	Botulism	Opioids
Nicotine	(cocaine)	Clonidine	Organophosphate
Organophosphate	Theophylline	Ethanol	Sedatives

Hyperthermia		Hypothermia
Amphetamines	Phencyclidine	Carbon monoxide
Anticholinergics	Phenothiazines	Ethanol
Arsenic (acute)	Salicylates	Hypoglycemic agents
Cocaine	Sedative-hypnotics	Opioids
Antidepressants	Theophylline	Phenothiazines
LSD	Thyroxine	Sedative-hypnotics

Mydriasis (pupillodilation)		Miosis (pupilloconstriction)	
Anticholinergics	Amphetamines	Anticholinesterase	Clonidine
Antihistamines	Cocaine	Opioids	Coma from barbit-
Antidepressants	Sympathomimetics	Nicotine	urates, benzodi-
Anoxia-any cause	Drug withdrawal	Pilocarpine	azepines, ethanol

Toxins that Cause Seizures[1]

Antidepressants	Cocaine, camphor	INH, Lead, Lithium	Organophosphate
β blockers	Ethanol withdrawal	PCP, theophylline	Sympathomimetics

[1] All agents causing ↓BP, fever, hypoglycemia and CNS bleeding can cause seizures.

Poisoning (Toxidromes)

Syndrome	Toxin	Manifestations
anticho-linergic	<u>Natural</u>: belladonna alkaloids, atropine, homatropine, amanita muscurina. <u>Synthetics</u>: cyclopentolate, dicyclomine, tropicamide, antihistamines, tricyclics, phenothiazines	<u>Peripheral antimuscarinic</u>: dry skin, thirst, blurred vision, mydriasis, ↑pulse, ↑BP, red rash, ↑temperature, abdominal distention, urine retention. <u>Central symptoms</u>: delirium, ataxia, cardiovascular collapse, seizures
acetyl-cholines-terase inhibition	insecticides (organophosphates, carbamates) Nerve gas agents (see page 17)	<u>Muscarinic effects</u> (SLUDGE): salivation, lacrimation, urination, defecation, GI upset, emesis. Also ↓or↑ pulse and BP, miosis. <u>Nicotinic effects</u>: ↑pulse, muscle fasciculations, weakness, paralysis, ↓respirations, sympathetic stimulation. <u>Central effects</u>: anxiety, ataxia, seizure, coma, ↓respiration, cardiovascular collapse
choli-nergic	acetylcholine, betelnut, bethanechol, clitocybe, methacholine, pilocarpine	see *muscarinic* and *nicotinic* effects above
extra-pyramidal	haloperidol, phenothiazines	<u>Parkinsonism</u>: dysphonia, rigidity, tremor, torticollis, opisthotonos
hemoglo-binopathy	carbon monoxide, methemoglobin	headache, nausea, vomiting, dizziness, coma, seizures, cyanosis, cutaneous bullae, "chocolate" blood with methemoglobinemia
metal fume fever	iron, magnesium, mercury, nickel, zinc, cadmium, copper	chills, fever, muscle pain, headache, fatigue, weakness
narcotic	morphine, dextromethorphan, heroin, fentanyl, meperidine, propoxyphene, codeine, diphenoxylate	CNS depression, miosis (except meperidine), ↓respirations, ↓BP, seizures (with propoxyphene and meperidine)
sympatho-mimetic	aminophylline, amphetamines, cocaine, ephedrine, caffeine, methylphenidate	CNS excitation, seizures, ↑pulse, ↑BP (↓BP with caffeine)
with-drawal syndrome	alcohol, barbiturates, benzodiazepines, cocaine, narcotics, opioids	diarrhea, mydriasis, piloerection, ↑BP, ↑pulse, insomnia, lacrimation, cramps, yawning, hallucinations

Poisoning Antidotes and Treatments

Toxin	Antidote	Other considerations
acetamino- phen	n-acetylcysteine see page 145 for dose	very effective if used within 8h, may be helpful up to 72h
β-blockers	glucagon 50-100 μg/kg IV, SC, or IM may repeat	glucagon may help reverse ↓pulse and ↓BP
Ca^{+2}channel blockers	CaCl$_2$ 45-90 mg/kg slow IV, or glucagon–see β blocker dose	glucagon may help reverse ↓pulse and ↓BP
cyanide	*Lilly Cyanide Kit* (see biologic & chemical agents page 17 for dosing)	Treatment induces methemo- globinemia & ↓BP. Sodium thiocyanate is excreted in urine.
digoxin	digoxin Fab fragments	see page 150 for dose
ethylene glycol	fomepizole (*Antizol*) 15 mg/kg IV, + 10 mg/kg IV q 12 h X 4	ethanol if *Antizol* not available, dialysis, see page 151 for detail
isoniazid	pyridoxine up to 50 mg/kg IV	reverses seizures
methanol	*Antizol*, dialysis, ethanol	See page 155 for detail
methemo- globinemia (nitrites)	methylene blue (0.2 ml/kg of 1% solution IV over 5 min)	consider exchange transfusion if severe methemoglobinemia
opiates	naloxone 0.1 mg/kg up to 2 mg IV	diphenoxylate and propoxyphene may require higher doses
organo- phosphates, carbamates	atropine 0.05 mg/kg IV pralidoxime (PAM)	exceptionally high atropine doses may be necessary, PAM doesn't work for carbamate toxicity
salicylates	dialysis, or sodium bicarbonate 1 mEq/kg IV	goal of alkaline diuresis is urine pH 7.50-7.55, see page 158
tricyclic anti- depressants	sodium bicarbonate 1 mEq/kg IV	goal is serum pH 7.50-7.55 to alter protein binding, see page 160

Radio-opaque Ingestions (CHIPES)
- **C**hloral hydrate and Chlorinated hydrocarbons
- **H**eavy metals (arsenic, Pb, mercury) health food (bone meal, vitamins)
- **I**odides, iron
- **P**otassium, psychotropics (e.g. phenothiazines, antidepressants)
- **E**nteric coated tabs (KCl, salicylates)
- **S**olvents (chloroform, CCl$_4$)

Drugs Cleared by Hemodialysis[1]
- Salicylates
- Ethylene glycol
- Methanol
- Bromide
- Isopropyl alcohol
- Chloral hydrate
- Lithium

Drugs Cleared by Hemoperfusion[1]
- Barbiturates (e.g. phenobarbital)
- Theophylline
- Phenytoin
- Possibly digoxin

[1] Consult local poison center for more detail concerning latest recommendations

HAZMAT (Hazardous Materials)
Phone numbers to ID hazardous chemical agents/spills and their management.
- CDC/Agency for Toxic Substances Disease Registry (ATSDR). (404) 488-7100
- Chemical Manufacturer's Association (CHEMTREC). (800) 424-9300

General Approach to the Poisoned Child

• Treat airway, breathing and BP	• Dextrose 10 ml/kg of D_{10} in neonate, 4 ml/kg $D_{25} \leq 2$ y, 2 ml/kg $D_{50} > 2$ y
• Insert IV and apply cardiac monitor	
• Apply pulse oximeter, administer O_2	• Administer naloxone 0.1 mg/kg

Charcoal

Initial dose is 1 g/kg PO or per NG mixed with cathartic

Contraindications	Drugs Cleared by Multi-dose Charcoal[1]
• Caustics (acids, alkalis)	theophylline, phenobarbital, digoxin,
• Ileus, bowel obstruction	propoxyphene, nadolol, phenytoin,
• Drugs bound poorly by charcoal (arsenic, bromide, K^+, toxic alcohols, heavy metals [iron, iodide, lithium])	diazepam, tricyclic antidepressants, chlorpropamide, nonsteroidals, and salicylates

[1] Administer repeat charcoal doses q 3-4 hours (use cathartic only for 1st dose).

Cathartics

Cathartics theoretically help by ↑ fecal elimination of charcoal-bound toxins, and preventing concretions. Monitor electrolytes closely with their use.	Cathartic choices
	• Sorbitol (35%) – 1 g/kg PO or NG
	• Magnesium citrate 4 ml/kg PO or NG
	• Na^+ or $MgSO_4$ – 250 mg/kg PO or NG

1 Only use cathartic one time (with 1st charcoal dose)

Ipecac

There are no absolute indications for use and some experts recommend never using in the ED. Ipecac delays charcoal administration, & has many adverse effects.

Gastric lavage

Directions for Lavage in Overdose	Indications
• Use 16-28 French *Ewald* tube	• Dangerous ingestion < 1 hour old
• Lavage stomach with 15 ml/kg NS aliquots until return is clear	• Toxins that slow GI transit
	• Toxins with possible rapid onset seizure, or ↓mental status
• Protect the airway with endotracheal intubation if there is an absent gag reflex, or altered mental status	• Toxins poorly bound by charcoal
	Contraindications
• Monitor total input and output from the *Ewald* tube	• Caustics (acids, alkalis), solvents (hydrocarbons), nontoxic ingestions

Whole bowel irrigation

Administration	Indications
• Place NG tube	• Iron, zinc, Li, sustained release meds
• Administer polyethylene glycol (*Go-Lytely*) at 25-40 ml/kg/h[1]	• Ingested crack vials or drug packets
	Contraindications
• Stop when objects recovered or	• CNS or respiratory depression
• Stop when effluent clear	• Ileus, bowel obstruction, perforation

1 until rectal effluent clear

Acetaminophen

Phase	Time after ingestion	Signs and Symptoms
1	30 min to 24 hours	Asymptomatic, or minor GI irritant effects
2	24-72 hours	Relatively asymptomatic, GI symptoms resolve, possible mild elevation of LFT's or renal failure
3	72-96 hours	Hepatic necrosis with potential jaundice, hepatic encephalopathy, coagulopathy, and renal failure
4	4 days - 2 weeks	Resolution of symptoms or death

Toxicity Assessment: ≥ 140 mg/kg (200 mg/kg) is potentially toxic. Obtain level ≥ 4h after ingestion & plot on nomogram. 4h level ≥ 140 µg/ml indicates need for n-acetylcysteine. On nomogram (below), level above dotted line (- - - - - -) = probable risk. Levels above bottom solid line (_____) = possible risk of toxicity. If unknown times, obtain level at 0 & 4 h to calculate T½ (if > 4h, give antidote).

Decontaminate	• Charcoal if toxic co-ingestant or waiting for drug level.
N-acetylcysteine *Mucomyst*	• If level will return < 8 h, delay treatment until level known. *Mucomyst* prevents 100% of toxicity if used < 8 hours from ingestion. If level will return > 8 hours and ≥140 mg/kg ingested, administer 1st dose. *Mucomyst* is definitely useful up to 24 hours after ingestion ± up to 72 hours. • Dose: 140 mg/kg PO, then 70 mg/kg PO q4h X 17 doses. • IV *Mucomyst* is used in Europe and not yet FDA approved.

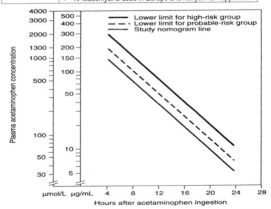

Used with permission. Copyright 1981 AMA. Rumack BH. *Arch Intern Med* 1981; 5: 871.

βeta-Blockers

<u>β1 stimulation</u> - ↑ contraction force + rate, AV node conduction, & renin secretion.
<u>β2 stimulation</u> - blood vessel, bronchi, GI, & GU smooth muscle relaxation.
Propanolol is nonselective, blocking β1 and β2 receptors. Other nonselective β-blockers: nadolol, timolol, pindolol. Selective β1 blockers: metoprolol, atenolol, esmolol, + acebutolol. Pindolol + acebutolol have some β agonist properties.

Clinical Features of β blocker overdose	
CNS	• Coma and seizures (esp. with lipid soluble agents – propanolol)
Cardiac	• ↓HR, AV block, ↑QRS width, ↑T waves, & ST changes
	• ↑HR with pindolol, practolol, and sotalol. ↓BP is common.
	• Congestive heart failure can occur.
Pulmonary	• Bronchospasm and respiratory arrest can occur.
Metabolic	• Hypoglycemia is more common in children compared to adults.

Treatment of β blocker Toxicity	
Option	Recommendations
Gastrointestinal decontamination	• Avoid ipecac. Aspiration & asystole are reported. • Charcoal - repeated doses, ± preceded by gastric lavage
Glucagon	• <u>Indications</u>: ↓HR or BP. • <u>Dose</u>: 50-150 µg/kg + 0.07 mg/kg/h IV
Atropine	• No HR response is suggestive of β-blocker toxicity. Administer 0.02 mg/kg IV prn (maximum of 0.5-1 mg).
Fluid/pressors	• If ↓BP does not respond to NS, administer α + β agonists (epinephrine/norepinephrine) or pure β agonists (dobutamine)
Other options	• Use pacemaker if no response to above. Consider dialysis if atenolol, nadolol, or acebutolol overdose. • Inamrinone – 0.75 mg/kg, + 5µg/kg/min IV (+inotropic effect)

Calcium Channel Blockers

System	Clinical Features
CNS	• Lethargy, slurring, confusion, coma, seizures, ↓respirations
Cardiac	• ↓HR, ↓BP, AV block (1st, 2nd or 3rd), sinus arrest, asystole
GI	• Nausea, vomiting, ileus, obstruction, bowel ischemia/infarction
Metabolic	• Hyperglycemia (esp. verapamil), lactic acidosis

Treatment of Calcium Channel Blocker Toxicity

Option	Recommendations
Gastrointestinal decontamination	• Charcoal ± preceded by gastric lavage. Avoid ipecac. • Whole bowel irrigation if sustained release preparation
Calcium	• Usually ineffective at improving cardiac conduction defects • Primary indication is to reverse hypotension • Administer Ca^{+2} gluconate 60-100 mg/kg IV over 5 minutes, repeat prn. Alternatively, CaCl$_2$ 20 mg/kg IV over ≥ 5 min.
Glucagon	• Indications: ↓HR or BP. • Dose: 50-150 µg/kg IV bolus + 0.07 mg/kg/h IV
Atropine	• Administer 0.02 mg/kg IV if symptomatic ↓HR (repeat X 3).
Fluids/pressors	• ↓BP occurs from peripheral vasodilation. Administer NS, then vasoconstrictors (e.g. norepinephrine, neosynephrine or ↑ dose dopamine).
Other options	• Use pacemaker if no response to calcium, glucagon, atropine.

Carbon Monoxide

Carbon monoxide (CO) exposure can occur from fire, catabolism of heme compounds, cigarettes, pollution, ice-surfacing machines, & methylene chloride (dermally absorbed

FIO$_2$	CO half-life
room air	320 min
100% rebreather	80 min
3 ATM hyperbaric O$_2$	23 min

paint remover) degradation. CO displaces O$_2$ off Hb shifting O$_2$-Hb dissociation curve to left. CO also binds cytochrome-A, cardiac and skeletal muscle myoglobin.

	Clinical Features
CO-Hb level	Typical symptoms at given level of CO toxicity
0-10%	Usually none, ±↓exercise tolerance, ↑angina, and ↑claudication
10-20%	Frontal headache, dyspnea with exertion
20-30%	Throbbing headache, dyspnea with exertion, ↓concentration
30-40%	Severe headache, vomiting, visual changes
40-50%	Confusion, syncope on exertion, myocardial ischemia
50-60%	Collapse, seizures
> 60-70%	Coma and death
Variable	Cherry red skin, visual field defect, homonymous hemianopsia, papilledema, retinal bleed, hearing changes, pulmonary edema. GI upset with vomiting (esp. common < 8 years old)

Assessment of CO Intoxication	
CO-Hb levels	Levels are unreliable & may be low in significant intoxication.
Anion gap	Cyanide and lactic acidosis may contribute to anion gap
Saturation gap	Calculated – directly measured arterial O2 saturation. This gap occurs with cyanide, methemoglobin, & sulfhemoglobin.
ECG	May show changes consistent with myocardial ischemia.
Cardiac enzymes	May be elevated from direct myocardial damage.

Treatment of CO Toxicity	
Criteria for Admission	**Criteria for Hyperbaric Oxygen**
• All with CO-Hb > 15-20% • Pregnancy and CO-Hb > 10% • Acidosis, ECG changes, myocardial ischemia, abnormal neurologic exam or history of unconsciousness • Symptoms after 100% O2 X 3h	• _Absolute_: cyanide toxic, coma, unconcious > 20 min, abnormal neurological exam, abnormal ECG, arrhythmias, or neurologic symptoms after 100% O2 X 3 h • _Relative_: pregnant, CO-Hb > 20%.

Clonidine

Clonidine is an α-adrenergic agonist with BP lowering properties, and ability to ameliorate opiate withdrawal symptoms. Tablets of clonidine (_Catapres_), in combination with chlorthalidone (_Combipres_), and transdermal patches (_Catapres-TTS_) are available. Used patches may contain up to 2 mg of active drug. Clonidine is rapidly absorbed from GI tract lowering BP within 30-60 min peaking at 2-4 h. Serum half-life is 12 h (6-24 h). Clonidine lowers BP at the presynaptic $α_2$-agonist receptors resulting in ↓ sympathetic outflow. At high doses, it is a peripheral α-agonist and causes ↑BP. It is also a CNS depressant.

Clinical Features	
General	• Up to 76% of children manifest symptoms by 1 h and 100% by 4h (unless sustained release pill). Symptoms usually last < 24h.
CNS	• Lethargy, coma, recurrent apnea, miosis, hypotonia
Cardiac	• Sinus bradycardia, hypertension (transient), later hypotension
Other	• Hypothermia and pallor

Treatment	
Monitor	• Cardiac monitor and pulse oximeter and observe closely for apnea. Apnea often responds to tactile stimulation.
Decontamination	• Charcoal ± gastric lavage. Avoid ipecac.
Atropine	• Indication: bradycardia. Dose: 0.02 mg/kg IV.
Antihypertensives	• Hypertension is usually transient. If needed, use short acting titratable agent (e.g. nitroprusside)
Fluids/pressors	• Treat hypotension with fluids and dopamine prn.
Naloxone	• 0.02 mg/kg IV may reverse CNS but not cardiac/BP effects.

Cocaine

Cocaine is the HCl salt of the alkaloid extract of the *Erythroxylon coca* plant. It can be absorbed across all mucous membranes. It is a local anesthetic.

Route	Peak effect	Duration
Nasal	30 min	1 – 3 hr
GI	90 min	3 hr
IV/Inhaled	1 - 2 min	≤ 30 min

(ester-type) that blocks the reuptake of norepinephrine, dopamine, & serotonin

Clinical Features of Cocaine Toxicity

General	• Agitation, hyperthermia, sweat, rhabdomyolysis, GI perf/ischemia
Cardiac	• A direct myocardial depressant, prolongs QT with sympathetic hyperactivity, myocardial ischemia (often with atypical clinical features & ECG findings - acutely or during withdrawal), ↑BP, ↑HR, LVH, arrhythmias, ↑platelet aggregation, accelerated atherosclerosis
CNS	• Seizures, CNS infarct or bleed, CNS abscess, vasculitis, dystonia
Lung	• Pneumothorax/mediastinum, hemorrhage, pneumonitis, ARDS

Management	
General	• Apply cardiac monitor, oxygen, pulse oximeter and observe for arrhythmia, seizures, and hyperthermia. Benzodiazepines are drug of choice for agitation, while haloperidol is also effective (without ↑ cocaine seizure threshold).
Hyperthermia & Rhabdomyolysis	• Benzodiazepines to reduce agitation and muscle activity. Cool with mist and fan. Continuous rectal probe temperature. Check serum CK/CO_2. Administer IV fluids & bicarbonate to prevent renal failure (page 40).
GI decontaminate	• *Body stuffers* – charcoal and monitor for perf./ischemia • *Body packer* – Xray and whole bowel irrigation. If rupture, consider laparotomy to remove cocaine
Cardiovascular (*Arrhythmias & Hypertension*)	• Administer benzodiazepines for ↑BP, ↑HR. Treat according to standard ALS protocols: Avoid β blockade (unopposed alpha). Use caution with labetalol:β > α block ± ↑ seizures. Use nitroprusside or phentolamine if severe HTN. • Wide complex tachycardia due to quinidine like effect. Give $NaHCO_3$ 1 mEq/kg IV & cardiovert. Avoid β blockers.
Cardiovascular (*Chest pain*)	• Administer benzodiazepines, aspirin, and IV NTG if MI. Phentolamine IV may reverse coronary vasoconstriction.
Neurologic	• Treat status epilepticus with benzodiazepines. Barbiturates are 2nd line while phenytoin is not useful. Exclude coexisting disease (CT, glucose, electrolytes, R/O infection).

Digoxin

Natural sources: foxglove, oleander, lily of the valley, and the "skin of toads".
Therapeutic range - 0.5-2.0 ng/ml. Severe poisoning may not demonstrate ↑levels.

Clinical Features – Acute Toxicity	
Digoxin level	Usually markedly elevated (obtain > 6 hours after ingestion)
GI and CNS	Nausea, vomiting, diarrhea, headache, confusion, coma
Cardiac	Supraventricular tachycardia, AV blocks, bradyarrhythmias
Metabolic	Hyperkalemia from inhibition of the Na^+/K^+ ATP pump

Clinical Features – Chronic Toxicity	
Digoxin level	May be normal
History	URI symptoms, on diuretics, renal insufficiency, yellow-green halos
Cardiac	Ventricular arrhythmias are more common than with acute toxicity
Metabolic	Potassium low or normal, magnesium is often low

Treatment of Digoxin Toxicity	
• Multi-dose charcoal ± lavage.	• ↑K^+: (page 47). Do not use calcium.
• Atropine 0.02 mg/kg for ↓HR	• Avoid cardioversion if possible (pre-
• Ventricular arrhythmia: lidocaine 1	disposes to ventricular fibrillation)
mg/kg IV ± $MgSO_4$ 25 mg/kg slow IV	• Digoxin Fab fragments (Digibind)

Indications for Digibind	Total body load digoxin - TBLD estimates
• Ventricular arrhythmias	TBLD (total body load of digoxin) in milligrams =
• Bradyarrhythmias	• [digoxin level[1] (ng/ml) x 5.6 x weight (kg)]÷1000
unresponsive to therapy	• or the total mg ingested if digoxin capsules or
• Ingestion of > 0.1 mg/kg	elixir is ingested
• Digoxin level > 5 ng/ml	• or the total mg ingested X 0.8 if another form of
• Consider if K^+ > 5.5 mEq/l	digoxin is ingested

[1] Chronic ingestions may have normal to mildly elevated digoxin levels.

Dosing Digibind
• Number of vials to administer = TBLD in mg divided by 0.5
• If ingested quantity unknown consider empiric administration of 2-10 vials
• One 38 mg Digibind vial can bind 0.5 mg of digoxin if amount ingested known
• Dilute Digibind to 10 mg/ml & administer IV over 20 min. Serum digoxin levels are useless after Digibind, as lab assay measures bound + unbound digoxin. These misleading levels may be exceptionally high, as Digibind draws digoxin back into the serum. Once bound, digoxin-Fab complex is renally excreted.

Ethylene Glycol

Ethylene glycol is found in coolants (e.g. automobile anti-freeze), preservatives, lacquers, cosmetics, polishes, and detergents.

Timing	Clinical Features
1-12 hours	• <u>Early</u>: inebriation, ataxia, slurring without ethanol on breath • <u>Later</u>: coma, seizures, and death
12-24 hours	• Cardiac deterioration occurs during this phase • <u>Early</u>: tachycardia, hypertension, tachypnea • <u>Later</u>: congestive heart failure, ARDS, & cardiovascular collapse • Myositis occasionally occurs during this phase
24-72 hours	• Nephrotoxicity with calcium oxalate crystal precipitation leading to flank pain, renal failure, and hypocalcemia

Diagnosis	Treatment
• Anion gap acidosis • Osmol gap[2] (measured – calculated osmol) > 10 mOsmL (page 44) • Hypocalcemia (ECG – ↑QT interval) • Calcium oxalate crystals in urine • ↑BUN and creatinine • Serum ethylene glycol level > 20 mg/dl is toxic • Serious toxicity has been reported in the <u>absence</u> of an elevated anion gap and crystalluria	• Gastric lavage (charcoal is ineffective) • NaHCO₃ 1 mEq/kg IV - keep pH ~7.40 • Ca⁺² gluconate 10%, 100 mg/kg IV if low calcium • Pyridoxine & thiamine IV • Fomepizole[1] (*Antizol*) – 15 mg/kg IV, + 10 mg/kg q12h X 4 doses, then ↑ to 15 mg/kg IV q12h until level < 20mg/dl • Dialysis if (1) oliguria/anuria, (2) severe acidosis, or (3) level > 50 mg/dl (> 20 mg/dl if fomepizole not used)

[1] Administer slow IV over 15 min. If unavailable, load IV ethanol (see Methanol).
[2] Osmol gap may be normal in significant toxicity.

Flunitrazepam - *Rophynol "Roofies"*

Rophynol is a benzodiazepine marketed outside the US for insomnia, sedation, & pre-anesthesia. It is 10 X as potent as diazepam. It potentiates and prolongs the effects of heroin, methadone, & alcohol and attenuates the withdrawal of cocaine. It produces disinhibition and amnesia and has been used as a "date rape" drug.

Onset/duration	• Maximal absorption is 0.5-1.5 hr with T½ of nearly 12 hours.
Major clinical effects	• <u>CNS</u> - sedation, incoordination, hallucinations. Paradoxical excitement, esp. with alcohol use. ↓DTRs, mid to small pupils. • <u>CV-Pulm</u> - Respiratory depression, hypotension, aspiration
Management	• NOT routinely detected in urine benzodiazepine screen • Lavage if < 1 h from ingestion, otherwise give charcoal • Protect airway and apply cardiac monitor, pulse oximeter • Admit if lethargic or unstable after 2-4 hr of observation.

Gamma Hydroxybutyric acid (GHB)

Gamma hydroxybutyric acid (GHB) has been promoted as a steroid alternative, a weight control agent, and as a narcolepsy treatment.

Onset/duration	• Onset of symptoms is ~ 15 minutes, with spont. resolution from 2 to > 48 hours (depending on dose & co-ingestant).
Major clinical effects	• <u>CNS</u> Acts with ethanol to produce CNS/respiratory depression. At ↑ levels patients are unresponsive to noxious stimuli & lose pharyngeal reflexes. Seizures, clonic arm/leg/face movements, vomit, amnesia, ↓DTRs, vertigo, nystagmus and ataxia occur. • CV-Pulm – ↓ HR, Irregular or ↓ respirations, ↓ BP.
Management	• Protect airway and apply cardiac monitor, pulse oximeter • Treat symptomatically (e.g. atropine for persistent ↓ HR). • Exclude coingestant or other diagnosis (e.g. CNS trauma) • Admit if symptoms do not resolve after 6 h of observation.

Iron Formulations	Elemental Iron	Mechanisms of Iron Toxicity
ferrous gluconate	12%	• Direct GI mucosal damage with hemorrhagic gastritis, bleeding
ferrous sulfate	20%	• Hepatic necrosis
ferrous fumarate	33%	• Mitochondrial damage
ferrous phosphate	37%	• Venodilation and hypotension
ferrous or ferric pyrophosphate	12%	• 3rd spacing of fluids
ferrocholinate	12%	• Thrombin inhibition- coagulopathy

Clinical Features – Staging of Iron Poisoning

Stage	Time post-ingestion	Findings
I	1-6 hours	Local toxicity: GI bleeding, perforation, diarrhea, and shock due to direct corrosion and vasodilation
II	2-24 hours	Relative stability and resolution: Stage I symptoms resolve
III	4-36 hours	Metabolic disruption: Metabolic acidosis, circulatory collapse, neurologic deterioration, hepatic failure, renal failure, coagulation defects, and third spacing of fluids.
IV	2-4 days	Liver failure: Hepatic necrosis
V	2-6 weeks	Late sequelae: GI tract scarring

Clinical Features – Suggestive of Iron Toxicity

• Vomiting and diarrhea (esp. ≤ 6h)	• Hypotension
• Mental status changes	• Coagulopathy, acidosis

Estimate of Quantity Elemental Iron Ingested and Toxicity Potential	Elemental Iron (page 152)	Toxicity
	< 20 mg/kg	None
	20-60 mg/kg	Mild to Moderate
	> 60 mg/kg	Severe

Serum Iron and TIBC levels

Obtain serum iron and total iron binding capacity (TIBC) at least 4 hours post-ingestion. Absorption and toxicity may be delayed for slow-release forms. Iron levels ≥ 350 µg/dl (normal 50-150) are serious, as the TIBC (350-500 µg/dl) may be exceeded. High iron falsely lowers TIBC measurements rendering this test unreliable.	Serum iron (µg/dl)	Toxicity
	< 100	None
	100-350	Mild
	350-500	Moderate
	500-1,000	Severe
	> 1,000	Possibly lethal

Adjunctive Diagnostic Tests

WBC count	> 15,000 cells/mm³ is associated with a serum iron > 300 µg/dl.
Glucose	> 150 g/dl is associated with a serum iron > 300 µg/dl.
KUB	Radio-opaque tablets on plain films indicate potential for further absorption/toxicity. 50% with iron > 300 µg/dl have negative X-ray.
Deferoxamine challenge	Test dose: 50 mg/kg IM. This agent binds free iron. After administration, pink or red urine indicates positive test. A negative test does **NOT** definitively exclude toxicity.

Treatment of Iron Poisoning

Fluid/blood	• Use NS ± blood prn. Consult surgeon if suspect perforation.
Decontamination	• Lavage with NS (esp. if iron on xray). Charcoal is ineffective.
Whole bowel irrigation	• Administer polyethylene glycol (*GoLytely*). (page 144). This option is especially useful if Xray shows tablets beyond pylorus.
Deferoxamine	• 15 mg/kg/h IV infusion. Do not wait for iron levels to return if the patient is symptomatic. Deferoxamine given IV or IM causes ↓ BP which is usually the limiting factor in infusion rate. Seizures can occur following deferoxamine. If improving, discontinue deferoxamine when urine clears and iron level <100 µg/dl.
Dialysis	• If renal failure prevents excretion of ferrioxamine

Indications for Chelation Therapy with Deferoxamine in Iron Toxicity	• Multisystem toxicity, eg, vomiting, diarrhea, GI bleeding, ↓BP, acidosis, altered mental status, coagulopathy
	• Tablets seen on plain abdominal radiograph
	• Positive deferoxamine challenge test
	• Serum iron > 350 µg/dl or serum iron greater than the TIBC (TIBC can be unreliable when serum iron levels are high)

Lead

A blood lead level (BLL) ≥ 0.48 mcmol/L (≥ 10 µg/dl) indicates ↑exposure in past. Risk factors: poverty, age < 6 y, inner city living, African-Am ethnicity. Lead may ingested (e.g. paint chips, old cans, lead coated products), inhaled, or absorbed (bullets or pellets). Early on, lead attaches to RBC then accumulates in bone. *Features* (1) <u>subclinical</u> (95% of cases)– accumulation of lead causes diminished cognition, altered behavior, shorter height, poor balance/coordination and hearing impairment. Children who live in or regularly visit a house built before 1950, or who live in or regularly visit house built before 1978 with recent or ongoing renovation (within past 6 months), or have siblings or playmates with lead poisoning are at risk (2) <u>clinical features</u> (only 5% are symptomatic). GI symptoms (anorexia, nausea, vomiting, intermittent pain, constipation) usually occur at a BLL threshold of 2.4 mcmol/L (50 µg/dl).although others develop symptoms as low as 0.97 mcmol/L or 20 µg/dl). CNS symptoms - developmental delay occurs (esp. speech delay). At BLL > 4.83 mcmol/L (100 µg/dl) encephalopathy occurs with altered mentation, ataxia, seizures, coma, ↑ICP. Heme – microcytic anemia, basophilic stippling. Bone - bands of density at long bone metaphyses [*lead lines*] (esp. distal femur, prox tibia/fibula).

Screening Recommendations by AAP and CDC		
If screening BLL is	CDC repeat venous blood lead level by	AAP repeat venous blood lead level by
0.48 – 0.92 mcmol/L (10-19 µg/dl)	3 months	1 month
0.97-2.12 mcmol/L (20-44 µg/dl)	7-28 days	1 week
2.17 – 2.85 mcmol/L (45-59 µg/dl)	48 hours	48 hours
2.90 – 3.32 mcmol/L (60-69 µg/dl)	24 hours	48 hours
≥ 3.38 mcmol/L (≥ 70 µg/dl)	Immediately	Immediately
Management Recommendations		
Diagnostic blood lead level (BLL)	CDC & AAP Action recommendations	
0.48 – 0.68 mcmol/L (10-14 µg/dl)	Repeat within 3 months	
0.72-0.92 mcmol/L (15-19 µg/dl)	Repeat within 2 months	
0.72-0.92 mcmol/L (15-19 µg/dl) on 2 tests or ≥ 0.97 mcmol/L (20 µg/dl)	Medical, nutrition, environmental Hx/PE with inspection, ± chelation, repeat BLL in 1 mo.	
2.17-2.85 mcmol/L (45-69 µg/dl)	As above, plus single drug chelation	
> 3.32 mcmol/L (> 69 µg/dl)	As above, plus double drug chelation	

Dosing of agents for lead toxicity can be complex & requires close monitoring. Options include EDTA, D-penicillamine, & DMSA.

Methanol

Methyl alcohol sources: wood alcohol, solvents, paint removers, shellacs, windshield washing fluids, and antifreeze. Toxicity is from formaldehyde/formic acid. Death has been reported after ingestion of 15 ml of 40% solution.

Clinical Features		Treatment
0-12 hours	• Inebriation, drowsiness • Asymptomatic period	• Gastric lavage (charcoal is ineffective) • NaHCO₃ 1 mEq/kg IV - keep pH >7.35
12-36 hours	• Vomiting, hyperventilation • Abdominal pain, pancreatitis • Visual blurring, blindness with mydriasis & papilledema • CNS depression	• Folate • Fomepizole (*Antizol*) – (see ethylene glycol dosing) • Ethanol (10%) in D₅W – (1) IV loading dose 10 ml/kg, (2) then 1.6 ml/kg/hour (3) Goal: ethanol level = 100-150 mg/dl
Diagnostic Studies		

• Osmol gap[1] may occur before anion gap acidosis (see page 44)
 • Anion gap and lactic acidosis
 • Hemoconcentration, hyperglycemia
 • Methanol levels > 20 mg/dl are toxic
   (1) CNS symptoms occur > 20 mg/dl
   (2) Visual symptoms occur > 50 mg/dl
		• Dialyze if (1) visual symptoms, (2) CNS depression, (3) level > 50 mg/dl, (4) severe metabolic acidosis, or (5) history of ingestion of > 30 ml.
		 • Stop dialysis and ethanol when methanol levels fall to < 20 mg/dl.

[1] Osmol gap may be normal in significant toxicity.

Mushrooms

Treat all toxic mushroom ingestions with IV fluids and GI decontamination. Specific antidotes are useful for certain classes of mushrooms as discussed below. Toxic mushrooms in groups I, II and VIII cause delayed symptoms (>6h from ingestion).

Phases of Cyclopeptide Mushroom Toxicity	Phase	Time	Features
	0	0-6h	asymptomatic latent phase (may last 24h)
	1	6-12h	gastrointestinal phase: vomiting, diarrhea
	2	12-24h	symptoms decrease, LFT's increase
	3	>24h	liver failure, shock, renal failure

Clinical Features, Onset, Treatment of Mushroom Toxicity

Group	Toxin	Onset	Symptoms	Treatment
I Cyclo-peptides	cyclopeptides amatoxins phallatoxins virotoxins	6-10h	See page 155	Multi-dose charcoal, IV NS, ± (penicillinG, cimetidine,thiotic acid, liver transplantation)
II MMH	monomethyl-hydrazine (MMH)	6-10h	CNS-seizures abdominal pain liver/renal failure	Pyridoxine ≥25 mg/kg IV, methylene blue for methemoglobinemia
III Muscarine	muscarine	½ - 2h	Cholinergic	Atropine
VI Coprine	coprine	½ - 2h	Disulfiram reaction (↑HR, flushed, vomit)	IV fluids
V Ibotinic acid and muscimol	ibotenic acid, muscimol	½ - 2h	GABA effects: (seizures, hallucinations), Anticholinergic	Benzodiazepines
VI Psilocybin	psilocybin psilocin	½ - 1h	Hallucinations (~LSD)	Benzodiazepines
VII GI toxins	multiple	½ - 3h	Pain, vomiting, diarrhea	IV fluids
VIII Orellines	orelline, orellanine	24 - 36h	Renal failure, vomiting	Supportive care, ± dialysis

Organophosphates and Carbamates

Organophosphates irreversibly bind and inhibit cholinesterases at CNS receptors, post-ganglionic parasympathetic nerves (muscarinic effects), and autonomic ganglia and skeletal myoneural junctions (nicotinic effects). Carbamates irreversibly bind cholinesterases and are less toxic.

Clinical Features of Insecticide Toxicity

Onset of symptoms	• Usually begin < 24h after exposure. Lipid-soluble organophos-phates (e.g. fenthion) may take days to produce symptoms with persistence for weeks to months and periodic relapses.
CNS	• Cholinergic excess: delirium, confusion, seizures, respiratory depression. Carbamates have less central effects.
Muscarinic	• SLUDGE (salivation, lacrimation, urination, defecation, GI upset, emesis), miosis, bronchoconstriction, bradycardia.
Nicotinic	• Fasciculations, muscle weakness, sympathetic ganglia stimulation (hypertension, tachycardia, pallor, rarely mydriasis)

Diagnostic Studies in Insecticide Poisoning

Labs	• ↑ glucose, ↑K+, ↑WBC, ↑amylase, glycosuria, proteinuria
ECG	• Early - ↑in sympathetic tone (tachycardia)
	• Later - extreme parasympathetic tone (sinus bradycardia, AV block, and ↑ QT)
Serum *(pseudo)* RBC *(plasma)* Cholinesterase	• Serum levels are more sensitive but less specific than RBC
	• Plasma levels return to normal before RBC levels
	• Mild cases: levels are < 50% of normal
	• Severe cases: levels are < 10% of normal

Treatment

General	• Support airway, breathing and blood pressure. Respiratory depression is the most common cause of death.
	• Medical personnel should gown and glove if dermal exposure.
	• Wash toxin off patient if dermal exposure.
	• Administer charcoal if oral ingestion.
Atropine	• Competitively blocks acetylcholine (Ach) at muscarinic (not nicotinic) receptors. Atropine may reverse CNS effects.
	• Dose: ≥ 0.05 mg/kg q 5 min. Mix 50 mg in 500 ml NS & titrate.
	• Goal: titrate to mild anticholinergic signs (dry mouth, secretions) and not to pupil size or heart rate.
	• Treatment failure most often due to not using enough atropine.
Pralidoxime (2-PAM)	• PAM has endogenous anticholinergic effects, while reversing nicotinic & central effects. It does not reverse carbamate toxicity.
	• Dose: 20-50 mg/kg IV over 15 minutes. May repeat q 10-12 hours. Onset of effect is 10-40 minutes after administration.
Atrovent	• Ipratropium bromide 0.5 mg nebulized q4-6h may dry secretions.

Salicylates

Methylsalicylate (oil of wintergreen) is the most toxic form. Absorption generally is within 1h of ingestion (delays ≥ 6h occur with enteric-coated and viscous preparations). At toxic levels, salicylates are renally metabolized. Alkaline urine promotes excretion. At different acidosis/alkalosis states, measurable salicylate levels change, therefore measure arterial pH at same time as drug level.

Ingestion	Severity	Signs and Symptoms
<150 mg/kg	mild	vomiting, tinnitus, and hyperpnea
150-300 mg/kg	moderate	vomiting, hyperpnea, diaphoresis, and tinnitus
>300 mg/kg	severe	acidosis, altered mental status, seizures, & shock

Clinical Features of Salicylate Toxicity

Direct	• Irritation of GI tract with reports of perforation
Metabolic	• <u>Early</u>: respiratory alkalosis from respiratory center stimulation • <u>Later</u>: anion gap acidosis - uncoupled oxidative phosphorylation • Hypokalemia, ↑or↓ glucose, ketonuria, and either ↑or↓ Na⁺
CNS	• <u>Early</u>: tinnitus, deafness, agitation, hyperactivity • <u>Later</u>: confusion, coma, seizure, CNS edema (esp. < 4 yo)
GI	• Vomiting, gastritis, pylorospasm, ↑ liver enzymes, perforation
Pulmonary	• Noncardiac pulmonary edema (esp. with chronic toxicity)

Indicators of Salicylate Toxicity

Clinical	• Features listed above are associated with toxicity
Ingestion	• Ingestion of ≥ 150 mg/kg is associated with toxicity
Ferric chloride	• Mix 2 drops FeCl₃+ 1 ml urine. Purple = salicylate ingestion
Phenstix	• Dipstick test for urine. Brown indicates salicylate or pheno-thiazine ingestion (not toxicity). Adding 1 drop 20N H₂SO₄ bleaches out color for phenothiazines but not salicylates.
Salicylate Levels	• A level > 30 mg/dl drawn ≥ 6h after ingestion is toxic. • Follow serial levels (q2-3h) until downward trend established. • In patients with a low pH, CNS penetration increases and toxicity can occur at lower levels. • *Done nomogram* may be unreliable indicator of toxicity.
Nontoxic Ingestion	• If none of the following are present, acute toxicity is unlikely (1) < 150 mg/kg ingested, (2) absent clinical features (3) level < 30 mg/dl obtained ≥ 6h after ingestion (unless enteric coated preparation, viscous preparation, or chronic ingestion)

Treatment

General	• Treat dehydration, electrolyte abnormalities. CSF hypoglycemia occurs with normal serum glucose – add D₅ or D₁₀ to all fluids.
Decontaminate	• Multi-dose charcoal. Whole bowel irrigation (if enteric coated).
Alkalinization	• Add 100 mEq NaHCO₃ to 1 L D₅½ NS (± 20-40 mEq/L K⁺ if no renal failure). <u>Goal</u> – urine pH > 7.5
Hemodialysis	• <u>Indications</u>: renal failure, noncardiogenic pulmonary edema, congestive heart failure, persistent CNS disturbances, deterioration of vital signs, unable to correct acid-base or electrolyte imbalance, salicylate level > 100 mg/dl (acutely)

Chronic Salicylate Toxicity

Presentation	• Patients are older, on chronic salicylates. Neuro changes & non-cardiogenic pulmonary edema are more common. Many are treated for infectious/neuro disease prior to correct Dx.
Toxicity	• Salicylate levels are often normal to therapeutic.
Treatment	• Supportive measures & urinary alkalinization are recommended. Dialyze if acidosis, confusion, or pulmonary edema.

Sympathomimetics (Amphetamines & Derivatives)

Effects of amphetamines are (1) <u>sympathomimetic</u> - α& β adrenergic - mydriasis, ↑HR, ↑BP, ↑temp., arrhythmias, MI, rhabdomyolysis, psychosis, CNS bleed, ↑sweat, seizures (2) <u>dopaminergic</u> - restlessness, anorexia, hyperactive, movement disorders, paranoia & (3) <u>serotonergic</u> – mood, impulse control, serotonin syndrome.

Ice/crank (crystal methamphetamine) 1 of most commonly synthesized illicit drugs. Onset is minutes, lasts 2-24 h. **MDMA – Ecstasy** – popular at "raves" and consumed orally. Low dose - euphoria, mild sympathomimetic symptoms last ~ 4-6 h. Potent serotonin releaser (no impulse control). High dose - effects (1-3) above.

Treatment (1) supportive care, cardiopulmonary & neuro monitoring, (2) anticipate complications, (3) benzodiazepines for agitation, (4) labetalol or nitroprusside– 1st line for ↑ BP (5) If ↓ BP, dopamine or norepinephrine (6) charcoal if oral ingestion, (7) treat MI, dysrhythmias, hyperthermia and rhabdomyolysis in standard fashion.

Theophylline

Clinical Features

Cardiovascular	• Tachycardia, atrial and ventricular dysrhythmias
Neurological	• Agitation, tremors, seizures
Metabolic	• ↑Glucose, ↑catecholamines, ↓potassium
Gastrointestinal	• Vomiting

Treatment

General	• Monitor for seizures, and arrhythmias. Correct dehydration, hypoxia, and electrolyte imbalances.
Charcoal	• Administer 1g/kg q2-4h. Repeat doses q4h.
Arrhythmias	• β-blockade is preferred for tachyarrhythmias (page 23-26). Do not use verapamil. It inhibits theophylline metabolism.
Seizures	• Use benzodiazepines (e.g. lorazepam) followed by barbiturates (e.g. phenobarbital). Phenytoin is *contraindicated*.
Hemoperfusion	• Indications (1) seizures, (2) poorly responsive arrhythmias, (3) theophylline level > 100 μg/ml in acute overdose or (4) theophylline level > 60 μg/ml in chronic overdose.

Tricyclic Antidepressants (TCA)

Clinical features are due to α adrenergic	ECG findings in TCA overdose
blockade ($\downarrow$BP), anticholinergic effects (altered mentation, seizures, $\uparrow$HR, mydriasis), inhibition of norepinephrine uptake (increasing catecholamines) and Na$^+$ channel blockade (causing quinidine like depressive effect on the heart). ^{1}ms – milliseconds; ^{2}bundle branch block	• Sinus tachycardia • $\uparrow$QRS > 100 ms[1], $\uparrow$PR interval, $\uparrow$QT interval, BBB[2] (esp. right BBB) • Right axis deviation of the terminal 40 ms of the QRS > 120 degrees • AV conduction blocks (all degrees) • Ventricular fibrillation or tachycardia (only occur in 4% who die from TCA's)

Treatment of TCA Toxicity

General	• Apply cardiac monitor, obtain ECG ✓QRS width, QT interval
Decontaminate	• Administer charcoal 1 g/kg PO or NG q2-4h. • Consider gastric lavage as anticholinergic effects may slow gastrointestinal transit. • Ensure patent airway & gag reflex prior to decontamination. • Avoid ipecac, as patients may have rapid mental status decline or develop seizures.
NaHCO$_3$	• <u>Indications</u>: (1) acidosis, (2) QRS width > 100 milliseconds, (3) ventricular arrhythmias, or (4) hypotension. • Alkalinization enhances TCA protein binding and reverses Na$^+$ channel blockade and toxic cardiac manifestations. • <u>Dose</u>: 1-2 mEq/kg IV. • <u>Goal</u>: Arterial pH of 7.50-7.55. • NaHCO$_3$ is ineffective for CNS manifestations (e.g. seizures)
Fluids/pressors	• Administer 10-20 ml/kg NS for hypotension. Repeat 1-2 X. • If fluids are ineffective administer phenylephrine or norepinephrine (not dopamine) due to prominent α effects.
Anti-seizure medications	• Use lorazepam followed by phenobarbital. • Phenytoin may be ineffective in TCA-induced seizures.
MgSO$_4$	• 25 mg/kg administered slow IV (over 15 minutes) may be useful for $\downarrow$ BP, and arrhythmias.
Disposition	*May transfer to psychiatric facility if all of following are present:* • no major evidence of toxicity during 6h ED observation • active bowel sounds • $\geq$ 2 charcoal doses are given • there is no evidence of toxic coingestant.

Trauma Scoring and Assessment

Pediatric Trauma Score[1]

Patient features	Score +2	Score +1	Score -1
Size (kg)	>20	10-20	<10
Airway	normal	maintainable	non-maintainable
Systolic BP (mmHg)	>90	50-90	<50
Mental status	awake	obtunded	comatose
Open wound	none	minor	major
Extremity fractures	none	closed	open or multiple

[1]A total score of ≤ 8 suggests possible serious injury, < 1 predicts mortality rate of >98%, 4 = 50% mortality, > 8 predicts < 1% mortality   *J Trauma 1988; 28:1038.*

Revised Trauma Score (RTS)[1]

RTS – add each category	Glasgow Coma Scale	Systolic BP	Resp. rate
4	13-15	> 89 mm Hg	10-29
3	9-12	76-89	> 29
2	6-8	50-75	6-9
1	4-5	1-49	1-5
0	3	0	0

[1] RTSC – modified for children – RR > 29 is normal (4) if aged 0-3 years; RTS < 12 indicates possibility of significant trauma, RTS < 7 = 79% probability of emergent surgery

Pediatric Glasgow Coma Scale[1]

Eye opening	Best motor	Best verbal
0-1 years	**0-1 year**	**0-2 years**
4. spontaneous	6. spontaneous movement	5. normal cry, smile, coo
3. to shout	5. localizes pain	4. cries
2. to pain	4. flexion withdrawal	3. inappropriate cry, scream
1. no response	3. flexion / decorticate	2. grunts
	2. extension / decerebrate	1. no response
	1. no response	
>1 year	**>1 year**	**2-5 years**
4. spontaneous	6. obeys	5. appropriate words
3. to verbal	5. localizes pain	4. inappropriate words
2. to pain	4. flexion withdrawal	3. cries or screams
1. no response	3. flexion / decorticate	2. grunts
	2. extension / decerebrate	1. no response
	1. no response	**>5 years**
		5. oriented
		4. disoriented but converses
		3. inappropriate words
		2. incomprehensible
		1. no response

[1]Total score indicates that injury is mild (13-15), moderate (9-12), or severe (≤ 8).

Initial Approach to Pediatric Trauma

Primary Survey (0-5 minutes)

Assessment	Action
Airway - assess air movement, while immobilizing cervical spine	Endotracheal intubate if (1) unable to ventilate, (2) altered mentation/aspiration risk, (3) need for hyperventilation in head injury, (4) flail chest, (5) severe shock See page 11-12 for ETT size and rapid sequence technique.
Breathing - assess ventilation effectiveness and oxygenation	Apply pulse oximeter (± end-tidal CO_2 monitor), O_2, perform needle thoracostomy for tension pneumothorax, occlusive dressing for sucking chest wound, and ETT if needed.
Circulation - assess strength, rate, quality of peripheral pulses, while stopping external bleed. See page 5 for complete list of normal vitals by age, weight, length. See pg 8-10 for central venous cath. sizes, & IO technique.	Attach cardiac monitor, apply pressure to external bleed, Assess peripheral pulse rate, quality, strength. Insert two large peripheral venous lines, and draw blood for type and crossmatch, and basic labs.
	<table><tr><th>Age</th><th>IV catheter size</th><th>Intraosseous size</th></tr><tr><td>0-1 year</td><td>20-22 gauge</td><td>17 Fr</td></tr><tr><td>>1-6 years</td><td>18-20 gauge</td><td>15 Fr</td></tr><tr><td>8-12 years</td><td>16-20 gauge</td><td>-</td></tr><tr><td>> 15 years</td><td>14-18 gauge</td><td>-</td></tr></table>
Disability - assess pupils and alertness (AVPU)	Assess pupils + Peds Glasgow Coma scale (pg 161), AVPU (**A**lert, responds to **V**oice, **P**ain, **U**nresponsive)
Exposure	Completely undress patient (begin radiant warming)

Resuscitation (Simultaneously Performed During Primary Survey)

Airway/Breathing	Reassess - see above
Circulation	Note: do not spend > 2-3 min attempting peripheral IV. If hypotensive, obtain IO or central venous access. Administer NS 20 ml/kg IV for hypotension/shock. Reassess, & repeat NS 20 ml/kg IV if needed. Administer 0 negative whole blood or packed RBC's 10-20 ml/kg. Insert NG tube, Foley catheter (see page 5 or 170 for size).

Secondary Survey and Definitive Care

Reassess ABCDE	Address any deterioration or new abnormalities. Insert chest tube prn (e.g. if prior needle thoracostomy).
Head to toe examination	Complete vital signs (do not forget back and rectal exams).
Address extremity injuries	Reduce dislocations compromising circulation.
Initial Xrays	Obtain cervical spine, chest, pelvis, extremity, CT scans.
Pain control, infection risk	Administer analgesics, antibiotics, tetanus.
Begin disposition	Call surgeon and consultants as need identified. Initiate transfer, admission, or prepare for operating room. Splint fractures and dress wounds
Documentation	Document all abnormalities (including xray, lab abnormalities), consults and times. Talk to family.

Abdominal Trauma

Independent Predictors of Intra-Abdominal Injury if Significant Pediatric Blunt Torso Trauma *Ann Emerg Med 2002; 39: 500.*	*Predictors[3]*	*Predictive Values* (95% confidence values)	
	• Low systolic BP	Sensitivity[1]	98% (93-100%)[2]
	• Abdomen tender	Specificity	49% (46-52%)
	• Femur fracture	Neg predictive value	99.6% (99-100%)
	• ALT > 125 U/L		
	• AST > 200 U/L		
	• Hematocrit < 30%		
	• UA with > 5 rbc/hpf	Pos predictive value	17% (14-20%)

[1] denotes sensitivity if any one of listed features present
[2] sensitivity for abdominal injury requiring surgery was 100% in this study.
[3] listed predictors + Glasgow coma scale < 14 = author's cited indicators for abdominal CT

Predictors of Abdominal, GU Injury, & Death Based on Pelvic Fracture Class

Torode class	Mortality	GU injury	Other Fx[2]	Neuro. injury	Abd surgery
II	0%	6%	39%	61%	11%
III	3%	26%	49%	57%	13%
IV	13%	38%	56%	56%	40%

[1] See page 118 for Torode Class   *J Pediatr Orthop* 1985; 5: 76. & 2002; 22: 22.
[2] Others found that multiple pelvic fx sites (80% associated injury) + a Revised Trauma Score (esp < 11, see page 161) predict abdominal/GU injuries. If only single fx site & a RTS of 11 or 12, only 0.5% intra-abdominal injury.   *J Trauma* 1991; 31: 1169.

Management of Blunt Abdominal Trauma

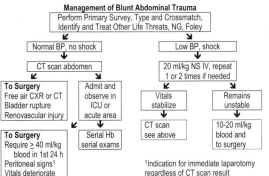

Head and Neck Trauma

See Independent Predictors of + CT scan & Intracranial Injury page 165.

Management of Minor Closed Head Injury (CHI) in Children ≥ 2 Years Old

Inclusion Criteria[1]	Exclusion Criteria[1,2]
• Age 2-20 years	• Age < 2 years
• Normal mental status upon exam	• Signs of skull fracture
• Normal neurologic examination	• Multiple trauma or spine injury
• May have LOC < 1 min, vomit, head-ache, or lethargy which resolved	• Unobserved loss of consciousness
• Evaluation within 24 hours of injury	• Bleeding diathesis underlying neuro. disorder (e.g. shunt, AVM)

Summary of American Academy of Pediatrics Recommendations	
Minor CHI, No LOC	• Observation in home, clinic, office or ED
	• CT, MRI, and skull radiography are not indicated
Minor CHI, brief LOC *(Asymptomatic)*	• Option 1 – observation (home, clinic, office, ED, hospital)
	• Option 2 – CT is acceptable
Minor CHI, brief LOC *(Symptomatic)*	• Signs of CHI (e.g. lethargy, repeat vomiting, ↑ headache)
	• CT scan

[1]Inclusion and exclusion criteria for use of parameter. [2]Does not imply mandatory imaging.

Pediatrics 1999; 104: 1407.

Management of Minor Closed Head Injury (CHI) in Children ≤ 2 Years Old [1,2]

High Risk	Intermediate Risk	Low Risk
↓Mental status	Vomit 3-4 times	*Additional risks:*	Low energy injury
Focal neuro. findings	LOC < 1 minute	↑ speed or force	(fall < 3 feet)
Basilar skull fx signs	Lethargy/irritability	ejected, fall >3-4 ft	No sign/symptom
Seizure or irritability	(now resolved)	Hematoma (esp non	> 2 h since injury
Acute skull fracture	Caretaker concern	frontal or large)	Age > 1 year is
Bulging fontanel	Non acute skull	Hard surface fall	reassuring if no
Vomiting ≥ 5X or > 6 h	fracture (> 24-48	Unwitnessed trauma	high or
LOC ≥ 1 minute	hours old)	Vague/no hx trauma	intermediate
	Age < 3-6 months	but signs/symptom	risks

High Risk	Intermediate Risk	Low Risk
CT scan	CT scan OR Observe 4-6 h	CT scan OR Observe 4-6 h	Discharge if
			No other injury
	If *additional risks* consider CT or skull radiography with CT if fracture found		No repeat vomit
			No altered LOC
			No abuse/neglect

Discharge only if negative CT, and if skull fracture present, it is simple and meets discharge criteria under low risk patients

[1] Guidelines do not cover birth trauma, penetrating injury, bleeding diathesis, shunt, multiple trauma, concern re: abuse/neglect, underlying neurologic disorder

[2] At this age scalp hematoma is 80-100% sensitive for skull fracture. The absence of skull fracture (& hematoma) and signs/symptoms of CHI has close to 100% negative predictive value for excluding significant intracranial injury. *Pediatrics* 2001; 107: 983.

Independent Predictors of A Positive CT Scan (+CT)[1] AND A Clinically Significant Intra-Cranial Injury (CS-ICI)[2] in 2043 Children < 18 Years	Predictors of a **+CT**	Predictive Values	
	• Altered mental status	Sensitivity	95.3%
	• Vomiting	Specificity	29.9%
	• Focal deficit	Neg pred value	98.6%
	• Scalp hematoma	Pos pred value	11.1%
	Predictors of a **CS-ICI**	Sensitivity	100%
	• Altered mental status	Specificity	47.8%
	• Vomiting	Neg pred value	100%
	• Headache	Pos pred value	8.8%

[1] Contusion, bleeding, or edema, [2] Required neurosurgical procedure, > 1 day admit, seizures meds > 1 week, or persistent neurologic deficit.

Pediatric Emerg Care 2002; 18:147.

Management of Increased Intracranial Pressure following Trauma

- Perform rapid sequence intubation while immobilizing cervical spine (pg 12).
- Keep pO_2 at least 90 mm Hg and pCO_2 at 35 mm Hg. (pCO_2 25-30 if herniating)
- Maintain normal BP and keep head of bed 30-45 degrees (if no spine fracture).
- Minimize stimuli such as pain, suctioning and movement.
- Consider mannitol 0.25-1.0 g/kg IV + sedative if hemodynamically stable.
- Consider anti-seizure meds (fosphenytoin PE - 15-20mg/kg IV < 2mg/kg/min) if

Glasgow Coma Scale < 9	Subdural hematoma	Large contusion
Delayed seizure	Depressed fracture with parenchymal damage	

- Keep ICP normal (15-20 mmHg).CPP (cerebral perfusion pressure) =MAP -ICP

| Differentiation of Accidental From Non-accidental Head Injury

Each listed feature differed significantly between groups		Abuse 6-7 months	Accident 2 ½ years
	Mean age	6-7 months	2 ½ years
	"Unwitnessed" injury	56%	2%
	Admitted assault	24%	0
	Motor vehicle	0%	23%
	Subdural hematoma	46%	10%
	Subarachnoid bleed	31%	8%
	Retinal hemorrhage	33%	2%
	Visceral injury	19%	4%
	Cutaneous injury	50%	16%
	Skeletal injury	35%	7%

Arch Pediatr Adolesc Med 2000; 154: 11-15

Sports-Related Concussion Grading

	Grade 1	Grade 2	Grade 3
Am. Academy of Neurology	• Brief altered mental status[1]	• Altered mental status > 15 min	• Any loss of consciousness
American College of Sports Medicine	• No loss of con-sciousness-LOC • Retrograde amnesia < 5 min	• LOC < 5 minutes • Retrograde amnesia > 30 min < 24 hours	• LOC > 5 minutes • Retrograde amnesia > 24 hours

[1] Difficult to recognize and may be briefly confused, or inattentive, or unable to perform a sequential task. *Pediatr Emerg Care* 2000; 16: 278.

American Academy of Neurology (AAN) &
American College of Sports Medicine (ACSM)
Recommendations to Return to Competition after Concussion[1]

	Grade[2,3]	AAN	ACSM
First Concussion	1	Same day	One week
	2	One week	One week
	3	2 weeks	Minimum one month with no symptoms for 1 week
Second Concussion	1	One week	2 weeks if no symptoms X 1 week
	2	2 weeks	Minimum one month with no symptoms for 1 week
	3	≥ 1 month (clinical decision of physician)	Season ending injury
Third Concussion	1	1 week	Season ending injury
	2	2 weeks	Season ending injury
	3	Season ending injury	Season ending injury

[1] Only if asymptomatic during exercise and while at rest. Sideline evaluation – check orientation, 4 digit recall, backward alphabet, memory testing (e.g. recall key game plays), brief sprint, pushups, sit ups. If headache, dizzy, unsteady, blurred vision, diplopia during exercise do not allow return to competition. Evaluate daily until symptoms resolve. Consider CT if symptoms ≥ 1 week, earlier if worsening.

[2] Grading is detailed on page 165.

Pediatr Emerg Care 2000; 16: 278.

NEXUS Criteria for Cervical Spine Imaging in Pediatric Blunt Trauma[1]

NEXUS criteria	Operator Characteristics[2] with 95% confidence intervals (CI)
Neck pain or midline tenderness	
Impaired consciousness, poor history	Sensitivity 100% (89-100%, 95% CI)
Neurologic deficit	Specificity 20% (19-21%, 95% CI)
Distracting/painful injury	Negative PV 100% (99-100%. 95% CI)
Intoxication	Positive PV 1% (1-2%, 95% CI)

[1] NEXUS Cspine study included 3065 patients < 18 y (88 < 2 years old, 817 - 2-8 years old, & 2160 - 8-17 years old). Criteria may not apply if < 2 years, trauma with underlying congenital/acquired spine instability (Down's, JRA, Klippel-Fiel syndrome, prior fracture)

[2] PV – predictive value   *Pediatrics* 2001; 108: e20.

Normal Cervical Spine spaces

A – Atlantal dens interval
(*Predental space*) < 5mm if <
8 y old, otherwise < 3mm.

B - *Posterior cervical line*, spino-
laminar line of C2 should be
within 2 mm anterior or
posterior to this line.

C - Prevertebral space ≤ 7 mm
in front of C2 or < 1/3 of
width of C2 vertebral body.

D - Limit of overriding of
vertebral bodies is 2.5 mm.

E - Retrotracheal space should
be < 14 mm in front of C6 or
< 5/4 of width of C5 in front
of C5 (# are inexact)

F - Prevertebral fat stripe -
should not bulge out.

X ÷ Y = *Power's ratio*
Normal value is 0.7 – 1.0
Value < 0.7 suggests
anterior subluxation of
atlantooccipital (AA) joint.

A line from the anterior margin of
the foramen magnum to the
tip of the odontoid should be
< 10-12 mm. If greater,
atlanto-occipital dislocation
may be present..

Wackenheim line – a line drawn
along posterior clivus usually
intersects tip of odontoid
tangentially. If displaced,
suspect atlantooccipital joint
laxity. May be unreliable in
young children.

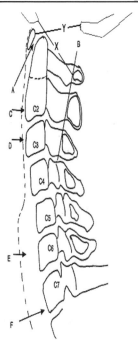

Used with permission –
Pediatr Emerg Med Reports 1996;1:83.

Cervical Spine Anatomy in Children < 8 Years Old
Normal lordosis to cervical spine is absent in 14% of children
Normal posterior angulation of odontoid seen in up to 4% of children
Majority of injuries occur at C1-C2 ≤ 8 years old and lower cervical spine > 8 years
Os odontoideum - congenital anomaly where odontoid does not fuse with C2[1]
Ossiculum terminale – A secondary center of ossification for odontoid tip, appears by age 3 (in 26% of children) and fuses with odontoid by 12 (may never fuse).
Prevertebral space at C3 is ≤1/3-2/3 of C3 vertebral body width or ≤ 5-7 mm[2]
Prevertebral space at C5 is ≤ 5/4 of (C5 or C6) vertebral body width or ≤ 14 mm[2]
Predental space up to 5 mm ≤ 8 years (up to 3 mm > 8 years)
Pseudo-Jeffersonian fx-C1 lateral masses grow faster than C2 so C1 overlaps C2 (usually < 6 mm). Present in 90% age 1-2, 18% aged 7 years.
Pseudosubluxation of C2/C3 or C3/C4 in 40% (normal variant where anterior aspect of C2 spinolaminar line is ≤ 2 mm ant or post to posterior cervical line(B on pg 167)

[1]spine injury with minor trauma occurs, [2] these norms can be unreliable in children

Development of Cervical Spine

Age	Feature
< 6 mo	C1 ring invisible and all synchondroses are open, vertebrate are normally wedged anteriorly, and there is often no lordosis to the un-injured spine
1 yr	body of C1 becomes visible radiographically
3 yr	posteriorly located spinous process synchondroses fuse dens becomes ossified (visible radiographically)
3-6 yr	neurocentral (body) and C2-odontoid synchondroses fuse summit ossification center appears at the apex (top) of the odontoid anterior wedging of the vertebral bodies resolve (now is not normal if seen)
8 yr	pseudosubluxation and predental widening resolve, lordosis tips is normal now
12-14	secondary ossification centers appear at spinous process tips (mistaken for fractures), summit ossification center of odontoid fuses (if it does not os odontoideum occurs), superior/inferior epiphyseal rings appear on body
25 yr	secondary ossification centers at tips of spinous processes fuse superior/inferior epiphyseal rings fuse to vertebral body

Spinal Cord Injury Without Radiologic Abnormality (SCIWORA)

SCIWORA accounts for 1/5 of all pediatric spinal cord injuries. Immediate plain films, CT are always normal, immediate MRI is normal in up to 50% with atrophy of spinal cord evident on MRI performed 1-3 mo after accident. Those with initial normal MRI almost always have 100% recovery. Delayed onset of neurologic deficit occurs in 54%, (mean 1-2 days) with half of the delayed onset complaining of paresthesias at the time of the accident. 83% of cases involve the cervical cord, and 2/3 are ≤ 8 years old. 44% have isolated sensory, 31% isolated motor, and 25% motor plus sensory deficits. For children with delayed paralysis, progression of weakness is rapid and usually causes complete cord lesion.

Clin Pediatr 1996; 119. *Am J Emerg Med* 1999; 17: 230; *Neurosurgery* 1994; 35: 406.

Spinal Cord Injury Syndromes[1], [2]

Anterior Cord Syndrome	Central Cord Syndrome
• Flexion or vertical compression injury to anterior cord or spinal artery	• Hyperextension injury
	• Motor weakness in hands > arms
• Complete motor paralysis	• Legs are unaffected or less affected
• Hyperalgesia with preserved touch and proprioception (position sense)	• Variable bladder/sensory dysfunction
• Loss of pain and temperature sense	• Prognosis is generally good and most do not require surgery
• Most likely cord injury to require surgery	**Brown-Sequard Syndrome**

Complete Cord Injury	Brown-Sequard Syndrome
	• Hemisection of cord
	• Ipsilateral weakness
	• Ipsilateral loss of proprioception
• Flaccid below injury level	• Contralateral loss of pain and temperature sensation
• Absent deep tendon reflexes	
• Decreased sympathetics	**Posterior Cord Syndrome**
• Warm skin, low BP, and slow HR	• Pain, tingling, of neck and hands
• Sensation may be preserved	• 1/3 have upper extremity weakness
• Priapism may be present	• Mild form of central cord syndrome
• If lasts > 24 hours, will be complete	

[1] diffuse flexion withdrawal can occur in children with paralyzed limbs if stimulation

[2] see page 98 for dermatomes and muscle testing.

Steroid Protocol for Treatment of Acute Spinal Cord Injury

- *Indications*: Acute spinal cord injury presenting within **8 hours** of injury.
- *Contraindications* (absolute and relative): Age < 13 y (many still treat), nerve root/cauda equina, gun shot, pregnant, on steroid, other life threatening illness
- *Protocol*: methylprednisolone 30 mg/kg IV over 15 min, then 45 min pause, then methylprednisolone 5.4 mg/kg/h IV over 23 h if < 3 h since injury OR over 47h if 3-8h since injury.   *New Engl J Med* 1990;322:1405;*JAMA* 1997;277:1597.

Renal and Genitourinary Trauma

Diagnostic Evaluation of Suspected Blunt Renal Trauma *J Urol* 1996; 2014.

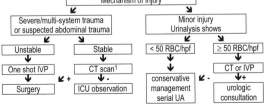

[1]CT-if multiple trauma, abdominal trauma, shock, pelvic, lumbar, thoracic or lower rib fracture. CT or IVP if minor trauma, or suspected ureteral injury (e.g. penetrating trauma).

Evaluation of Suspected Urethral Trauma

Retrograde Urethrogram Indications	Retrograde Urethrogram Technique
Penile, perineal, vaginal or scrotal trauma	Obtain preinjection KUB film
Blood at urethral meatus or cannot void	Place Cooke adapter or Christmas tree
Extravasation of blood/urine to scrotum, perineum, abdominal wall or penile shaft	adapter on end of 30-60 ml syringe. (may substitute Foley - see below)
Abnormal prostate examination	Inject 0.2 ml/kg of contrast dye over 60
Significant pelvic fracture	seconds
Inability to easily pass Foley catheter	Take xray during last 10 seconds

Evaluation of Suspected Bladder Trauma

Cystogram Indications	Cystogram Technique
Penetrating injury to low abdomen or pelvis	After urethrogram empty bladder
Blunt lower abdominal-perineal trauma with significant microscopic hematuria (> 20 RBC/ hpf), gross blood, blood at meatus	Instill contrast into bladder until 5ml/kg or discomfort or bladder is full (see formula below for normal bladder volume)
Significant pelvic fracture	Obtain oblique, and AP films of bladder,
Unable to void or minimal urine after Foley	empty bladder then repeat films.

Bladder volume if [< 1 yr = weight (kg) X 10 ml]; if [≥ 1 yr =(age in years + 2) x 30 ml]

Estimated Urethral Catheter Size (French) Based on Age (Years)

Age	1 day	3 mo	1	3	6	8	10	12	teen
Size	5	8	8-10	10	10	10-12	12	12-14	16+

Thoracic Trauma

Independent Predictors of Intra-Thoracic Injury if Significant Pediatric Blunt Torso Trauma *Ann Emerg Med 2002; 39: 492.*	*Predictors*	*Predictive Values* (95% confidence values)	
	• ↓BP or ↑ resp rate	Sensitivity[1]	98% (91-100%)[2]
	• Chest wall tender abraded/contused	Specificity	37% (34-40%)
	• ↓Breath sounds or rales or rhonchi	Neg predictive value	99% (98-100%)
	• Femur fracture	Pos predictive value	12% (10-15%)
	• GCS < 15		

[1] Sensitivity if any one of identified predictors is present. [2] 100% sensitive in predicting abnormality requiring therapy in this single study.

Rib Fracture Etiology In Infants < 1 year	Abuse	82%	Fragile bones	8%
	Nonintentional	8%	Birth trauma	3%

[1] Includes osteogenesis imperfecti, rickets, prematurity.

Chest tube sizes (French) for Hemothorax/Pneumothorax Based on Age

Age	1mo	0.5	1	3	5-6	8	12	16
Size	12-18	14-20	14-24	16-28	20-32	24-32	28-36	28-40

Emerg Med Clin North Am 1993; 11: 187.

Genital Disorders - Male

The Painful Scrotum

Feature	Torsion of Testicle	Epididymitis & Orchitis	Torsion of Testicular Appendix
Frequency, age 0-20 yr	25-50%	10-25%	30-50%
Frequency, age 20-29	20%	80%	0%
Pain onset	acute onset	gradual onset	gradual onset
Pain location	testis, groin, abdomen	testes, groin, epididymis	testis or upper pole
Prior similar episodes	often	rare	rare
Fever	rare	up to 1/3	rare
Dysuria	rare	common	rare
Testicle/Scrotum	horizontal high riding testis	firm, red, warm scrotum (>70%)	usually nontender, blue-dot upper testis
Cremasteric reflex	usually absent	may be present	may be present
Pyuria	up to 10%	25-60%	rare
Doppler / Nuclear scan	↓ flow	↑ flow	normal flow

Evaluation

- Contact urologist immediately if torsion suspected. Immediate surgical exploration has best chance of saving testicle. If clinical suspicion is low, consider one of diagnostic tests below after consultation with urologist.
- Doppler has 80-90% sensitivity and specificity in diagnosing testicular torsion. Absent flow is suspicious for torsion while intact flow suggests inflammation. Perform funicular compression during Doppler: Compress the testicular artery to see if flow stops. This signifies Doppler flow was testicular, not scrotal.
- Nuclear scan is ~85% sensitive & > 95% specific for torsion. False negative exams occur if small testicles (infants), spontaneous detorsion, or early torsion.
- Color doppler flow is 86-100% sensitive and 100% specific for torsion in adults.

Pediatr Clin North Am 1997; 44: 1065.

If ≥ 3 of the 6 *Knight and Vassey* criteria were present, risk of testicular torsion risk was 0 in study. In this study, no torsion cases occurred in 395 children who had ≥ 3 criteria, while all 130 confirmed testicular torsion cases had < 3 criteria. Furthermore, the presence of a *cremasteric reflex* almost always excludes torsion, although its absence is not specific for any disorder.

Knight and Vassey Criteria
• Gradual pain onset
• Dysuria, urethral discharge, recent cystoscopy, or indwelling Foley
• History of UTI, imperforate anus, hypospadias, or bladder dysfunction
• Temperature > 101 F
• Tender/indurated epididymis
• > 10 WBC/high power field in urine
Knight, Vassey. *Ann Surg* 1984; 200: 664

OUTPATIENT PEDIATRIC DRUGS		*Age*	*2m*	*4m*	*6m*	*9m*	*12m*	*15m*	*2y*	*3y*	*5y*
		Kg	5	6½	8	9	10	11	13	15	19
		Lbs	11	15	17	20	22	24	28	33	42
med	***strength***	***freq***	***teaspoons of liquid per dose*** *(1 tsp= 5 ml)*								
Tylenol (milligrams)		q4h	80	80	120	120	160	160	200	240	280
Tylenol (tsp)	160/t	q4h	½	½	¾	¾	1	1	1¼	1½	1¾
ibuprofen (milligrams)		q6h	-	-	75†	75†	100	100	125	150	175
ibuprofen (tsp)	100/t	q6h	-	-	¾†	¾†	1	1	1¼	1½	1¾
amoxicillin or	125/t	bid	1	1¼	1½	1¾	1¾	2	2¼	2¾	3½
Augmentin	200/t	bid	½	¾	1	1	1¼	1¼	1½	1¾	2¼
regular dose	250/t	bid	½	½	¾	¾	1	1	1¼	1¼	1¾
	400/t	bid	¼	½	½	½	¾	¾	¾	1	1
amoxicillin or	200/t	bid	--	1¼	1½	1¾	2	2¼	2½	3	4
Augmentin	250/t	bid	--	1¼	1½	1½	1¾	1¾	2¼	2½	3
high OM dose‡	400/t	bid	--	¾	¾	1	1	1¼	1½	1½	2
Augmentin ES‡	600/t	bid	--	½	½	¾	¾	¾	1	1¼	1½
azithromycin*§	100/t	qd	--	½†	½	½	½	½	¾	¾	1
"	200/t	qd	--	¼†	¼	¼	¼	¼	½	½	½
Bactrim/Septra	---	bid	½	¾	1	1	1	1¼	1½	1½	2
cefaclor*	125/t	bid	--	1†	1¼†	1½	1½	1¾	2	2½	3
"	250/t	bid	--	½†	¾†	¾	¾	1	1	1¼	1½
cefadroxil	125/t	bid	½	¾	1	1	1¼	1¼	1½	1¾	2
"	250/t	bid	¼	½	½	½	¾	¾	¾	1	1
cefdinir	125/t	qd	--	¾†	1	1	1	1¼	1½	1¾	2
cefixime	100/t	qd	--	½	¾	¾	¾	1	1	1¼	1½
cefprozil*	125/t	bid	--	¾†	1	1	1¼	1½	1½	2	2¼
"	250/t	bid	--	½†	½	½	¾	¾	¾	1	1¼
cefuroxime	125/t	bid	½	¾	¾	1	1	1	1¼	1½	2
cephalexin	125/t	qid	--	½†	¾†	¾†	1	1	1¼	1½	1¾
"	250/t	qid	--	¼†	¼†	½†	½	½	¾	¾	1
clarithromycin	125/t	bid	--	½†	½†	½	¾	¾	¾	1	1¼
"	250/t	bid	--	¼†	¼†	¼	½	½	½	½	¾
dicloxacillin	62½/t	qid	½	¾	1	1	1¼	1¼	1½	1¾	2
loracarbef*	100/t	bid	--	1†	1¼	1½	1½	1¾	2	2¼	3
nitrofurantoin	25/t	qid	¼	½	½	½	½	¾	¾	¾	1
Pediazole	---	tid	½	½	¾	¾	1	1	1	1¼	1½
penicillin	125/t	qid	½	½	¾	¾	1	1	1¼	1¼	1½
"	250/t	qid	--	¼	¼	½	½	½	¾	¾	1
Benadryl	12.5/t	q6h	½	½	¾	¾	1	1	1¼	1½	2
Dimetapp	---	q4h	-	-	¼†	¼†	½	¾	¾	1	1
prednisolone	15/t	qd	¼	½	½	¾	¾	¾	1	1	1¼
prednisone	5/t	qd	1	1¼	1½	1¾	2	2¼	2½	3	3¾
Robitussin	---	q4h	-	-	¼†	¼†	½	½	¾	¾	1
Rondec	---	q4h	-	-	-	-	¼†	¼†	½	½	1
Triaminic	---	q4h	-	¼	¼	¼	½	½	1	1	1
Tylenol w/ Codeine		q4h	-	-	-	-	-	-	-	1	1
Ventolin	2/t	tid	-	-	-	-	½	½	¾	¾	1
Zyrtec	5/t	qd	-	-	-	-	-	-	½	½	½

* Dose is for otitis media only;† Dosing at this age/weight not recommended by manufacture
‡ ↑ dose (80-90 mg/kg/d) is for otitis media if ↑ risk for penicillin-resistant *S pneumoniae* (ag
<2 yo, antibiotics within ≤ 3 months, day care).§Give double dose of azithromycin 1st day

Critical Drugs & IV Infusions

Detail regarding indications, dosing, side effects, contraindications are listed for Resuscitation (page 5-10), Cardiovascular (22-26), HTN (71-73), Seizures (102)

Adenosine	• 0.05-0.1 mg/kg IV (maximum dose 6 mg), may double to 0.3 mg/kg (maximum dose 12 mg)
Amiodarone	• 5 mg/kg IV bolus if pulseless VT/VF, over 20-60 min if perfusing rhythm. May repeat up to maximum of 15 mg/kg/day
Atropine	• 0.01-0.02 mg/kg IV (minimum dose 0.1 mg, maximum 0.5 mg)
Diazepam	• 0.1-0.3 mg/kg IV (max dose 5 mg) or 0.5 mg/kg PR
Dobutamine	• 0.5-25 microg/kg/min (0.5-3.0: renal, mesenteric; 5-10: inotropic [cardiac output]; > 10 alpha adrenergic – ↑ BP, ↑ HR)
Dopamine	• 2-20 microg/kg/min IV
Enalaprilat	• 5-10 microg/kg IV
Epinephrine	• APLS: 0.01 mg/kg IV q 3-5 min; infusion: 0.1-1.0microg/kg/min
Esmolol	• 0.5 mg/kg IV over 1 min, then 0.05-0.25 mg/kg/min
Fosphenytoin	• 15-20 mg/kg (PE) IV @ < 2 mg/kg/min or IM
Isoproterenol	• 0.05-1.0 microg/kg/min IV
Labetalol	• 0.2-0.5 mg/kg IV (max 20 mg), then 0.25-1.5 mg/kg/hour
Lidocaine	• 1 mg/kg IV; infusion: 20-50 microg/kg/min
Lorazepam	• 0.05-0.1 mg/kg IV (max single dose 4 mg)
Midazolam	• 0.1-0.2 mg/kg IV/IM then 1-10 microg/kg/min(status epilepticus)
Nitroprusside	• 1.0-8.0 microg/kg/min IV
Norepinephrine	• 0.1-2.0 microg/kg/min IV
Phenobarbital	• 15-20 mg/kg IV (may ↑ to total 30 mg/kg in select cases)
Phenylephrine	• 5-20 microg/kg IV q 10-15 min OR 0.1-0.5 microg/kg/min
Procainimide	• 15 mg/kg IV over 30-60 min, stop if ↓ BP, ↑ QRS 50%,
Prostaglandin E1	• 0.05-0.10 microg/kg/minute (failure to respond, may mean ductus, pulm. venous return obstruction). Side effects: apnea, seizures, ↓BP, ↓ glucose/Ca, sepsis, diarrhea, NEC, renal failure, bleed.
Verapamil	• 0.1 mg/kg IV (max 5 mg). Repeat 0.2 mg/kg (max 10mg) in 30 min if no effect. Do not use < 1 year old and exercise caution if 1-8 year old age.

Ordering Books From Tarascon Publishing

FAX	**PHONE**	**INTERNET**	**MAIL**
Fax credit card orders 24 hrs/day toll free to **877.929.9926**	For phone orders or customer service, call **800.929.9926**	Order through our OnLine store with your credit card at **www.tarascon.com**	Mail order & check to: **Tarascon Publishing** PO Box 1159 Loma Linda, CA 92354

Name

Address

City		State	Zip

Please send me:	Number	Price ‡
Tarascon Pocket Pharmacopoeia, Classic Shirt-Pocket Edition		$
Tarascon Pocket Pharmacopoeia, Deluxe Labcoat Pocket Edition		$
Tarascon Pediatric Emergency Pocketbook		$
Tarascon Adult Emergency Pocketbook		$
Tarascon Internal Medicine & Critical Care Pocketbook		$
Tarascon Pocket Orthopaedica		$
How to be a Truly Excellent Junior Medical Student		$
Sheet Magnifier – Fits in any book to make reading easier!		$

‡ Price per Copy by Number of Copies Ordered					Subtotal	$
Total # of each ordered	1–9	10–49	50–99	≥100		
Pocket Pharmacop Classic	$ 8.95	$ 7.95	$ 6.95	$ 5.95		
Pocket Pharmacop Deluxe	$17.95	$15.25	$13.45	$12.55		
Peds Emerg Pocketbook	$11.95	$ 9.90	$ 8.95	$ 8.35	California	$
Adult Emerg Pocketbook	$11.95	$ 9.90	$ 8.95	$ 8.35	only add	
Internal Med Pocketbook	$11.95	$ 9.90	$ 8.95	$ 8.35	7.75%	
Pocket Orthopaedica	$11.95	$ 9.90	$ 8.95	$ 8.35	sales tax	
How…Truly Excellent JMS	$ 9.95	$ 8.25	$ 7.45	$ 6.95	Shipping	$
Sheet Magnifier	$ 1.00	$ 0.89	$ 0.78	$ 0.66	and	

Shipping & Handling				handling (table)	
If subtotal is →	<$10	$10-29	$30-75	$76-300	
Standard shipping	$ 1.00	$ 2.50	$ 6.00	$ 8.00	$
UPS 2-day air*	$12.00	$14.00	$16.00	$18.00	**TOTAL**

*No post office boxes

☐ **Charge credit card**: ☐ VISA ☐ Mastercard ☐ AmEx ☐ Discover

Card number		Exp Date
Signature	E-mail	Phone